Physiology and Pathology of the Mucociliary System

Advances in Oto-Rhino-Laryngology

Vol. 43

Series Editor
C.R. Pfaltz, Basel

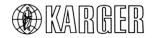

Basel · München · Paris · London · New York · New Delhi · Singapore · Tokyo · Sydney

Physiology and Pathology of the Mucociliary System

Special Regards to Mucociliary Transport in Malignant Lesions of the Human Larynx

Th. Deitmer, Münster

34 figures, 50 diagrams, 2 color plates and 3 tables, 1989

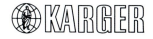

KARGER

Basel · München · Paris · London · New York · New Delhi · Singapore · Tokyo · Sydney

Advances in Oto-Rhino-Laryngology

Library of Congress Cataloging-in-Publication Data
Deitmer, Th. (Thomas), 1954-
Physiology and pathology of the mucociliary system: special regards to mucociliary transport
in malignant lesions of the human larynx/Th. Deitmer.
(Advances in oto-rhino-laryngology; vol. 43)
1. Mucociliary system-Pathophysiology. 2. Mucociliary system-Physiology.
3. Larynx-Tumors-Pathophysiology. I. Title. II. Series.
[DNLM: 1. Cilia-pathology. 2. Cilia-physiology. 3. Larynx-pathology.
4. Mucociliary Clearance. 5. Mucus-pathology. 6. Mucus-physiology.
ISBN 3-8055-4944-X

Bibliographic Indices
This publication is listed in bibliographic services, including Current Contents® and Index Medicus.

Drug Dosage
The author and the publisher have exerted every effort to ensure that drug selection and dosage set forth in this text are in accord with current recommendations and practice at the time of publication. However, in view of ongoing research, changes in government regulations, and the constant flow of information relating to drug therapy and drug reactions, the reader is urged to check the package insert for each drug for any change in indications and dosage and for added warnings and precautions. This is particularly important when the recommended agent is a new and/or infrequently employed drug.

Contents

Contents   VII

Acknowledgements

First of all I wish to express my sadness at the sudden death of Professor Dr. Fromme of the Institute of Medical Physics. He gave me much personal encouragement with electron microscopy. I also wish to thank his colleagues, Frau Dr. Pfautsch, Frau Dr. Grote and Frau Malkus.

I wish to thank the following:

Professor Dr. Feldmann, Director of the University ENT Clinic, for the important stimulus and discussion of this work.

Professor Dr. Guelker, Privatdozent Dr. Thale (University Medical Clinic) and Drs. Reers, Ruland and Spiegel (University Surgical Clinic) for co-operation and kind permission to take part in animal experiments.

Apotheker Duda (Pharmacist in the University Clinic) and Professor Dr. Thiem (Institute for Organic Chemistry of the University) for help with pharmaceutical problems and with preparation of a marker substance, respectively.

Dr. Reisch of the Institute for Biomathematics and Medical Informatics of the University for help with mathematical problems.

Professor Dr. Richrath of the University ENT Clinic for much help with the method and technical matters.

Professor Dr. E. Grundmann of the Gerhard Domagk Institute for Pathology of the University of Münster for help with the preparation and histology of specimens of laryngeal carcinoma.

All my colleagues at the University ENT Clinic who were so helpful during the execution of the clinical investigations.

I am indebted to Professor Dr. P.M. Stell for the translation and to the Deutsche Gesellschaft für Hals-Nasen-Ohrenheilkunde, Kopf- und Halschirurgie for financial support.

Foreword

The ancient Greek philosopher Heraklit (about 500 B.C.) framed his profound insight into the fundamental mechanism governing Nature and the Universe in his statement 'panta rhei': everything is flowing, nothing is at rest. Flowing means that some material is transported from one place to the other, and transportation, in fact, seems to be one of the essential processes by which the physiological equilibrium is maintained, carrying materials and messages, and weaving innumerable places and reactions into the pattern of a living individual.

We find transportation at the level of cells in the dimension of atoms and molecules governed by physical processes like diffusion and osmosis, or by active biological processes like secretion and absorption. The nervous system transports electrical and chemical signals, handling an enormous flow of information. In other organ systems there is mass transportation of various materials driven by muscular action: heart and blood circulation, carrying metabolic building blocks, hormones, heat and a multitude of other things; intestines and peristalsis conveying ingesta; inspiratory muscles transporting gases, vapors and airborne particles.

There is a special system of transportation for dealing with the airborne particles, contaminating the air we breathe. It is continually cleansing and renovating the surfaces of the respiratory system: the mucociliary apparatus. From a phylogenetic point of view this system combines two of the very earliest achievements of Nature, the production of mucus, which is already present in primitive algae, and the principles of locomotion or transportation by the whipping movement of cilia, realized to perfection already in certain protozoa.

This book gives an excellent survey of our knowledge of the mucociliary transport in the respiratory system, based on a thorough evaluation of the literature and the author's own investigations. Defects of this transporting mechanism may be due either to malproduction of the mucus or to malfunction of the ciliary apparatus. They are the root cause of manifold diseases of the respiratory system. The author's own studies demonstrate that inhaled particles, carcinogenic as they may be, are transported by the mucociliary system from the bronchi via the trachea to the sublaryngeal region, where they have to by-pass the non-ciliated vocal cords in order to get drained into the alimentary tract. Larynges that had developed carcinoma regularly show abnormalities of the mucociliary transport in this region.

It is my pleasure to introduce this book to the reader. It will certainly contribute considerably to our understanding of the pathophysiology of diseases of the respiratory system, including nose and sinuses, larynx, trachea, and bronchi, be they inborn or acquired, inflammatory, acute or chronic, traumatic or neoplastic. Thus it will prove a valuable source of information for all specialists involved in the treatment of these diseases.

Professor Dr. *Harald Feldmann*
Director of the ENT Department of
the University of Münster

1. Introduction

Examination of the human nasal cavity or endoscopy of the trachea and bronchi seldom reveals the existence of a lining by ciliated epithelium or even the physiological necessity for it. Because of their function these hollow spaces are unsuitable for cleaning by peristalsis. Lining of the walls by a self-cleaning carpet is thus a satisfactory phylogenetical solution [345].

An industrial worker in a dusty atmosphere, or the exhaust of a central heating plant which is not continually cleaned, provide impressive evidence of the need for permanent cleaning of the air. It is easy to imagine the environmental stress placed on the mucosa of the human airways if this continuous but invisible cleaning mechanism functions poorly. The conclusion that many respiratory diseases have their origin in an excess burden of inhaled toxins is inescapable. A slight disturbance of this clearance mechanism may prepare the way for various diseases. A typical example is the high proportion of smokers amongst patients with bronchial and laryngeal carcinoma.

Laryngeal carcinoma, the commonest tumour of the ear, nose and throat, arises at a point where the ciliary transport pathways of the bronchial system converge. It is well known that laryngeal carcinoma is caused by inhaled noxious agents. Since the mucociliary clearing system should protect against such noxious agents, or carry away the injurious substances, it is worthwhile investigating the role of lesions of the mucociliary system in laryngeal carcinoma.

A detailed analysis of this ciliary cleansing mechanism thus promises to yield basic knowledge about pathogenetic processes. The methods of investigation should provide data about both morphology and function. Observation of the function of the cilia, the basic functional elements of this cleansing mechanism, carries a certain aesthetic satisfaction.

A review of the current knowledge in this area will be provided before my own methods of investigation and results are described.

2. Historical Review

The discovery of the cilia was made possible by the development of the microscope; Antweiler [24] tells us that Johannes Ham, a student at Leiden, was the first to observe ciliary movements in man in 1677. This discovery was then confirmed by Van Leeuwenhoek in seminal fluid. The existence of a ciliary epithelium in mussels was discovered in 1684 by Antonius de Heide [168] in the Netherlands.

However it was not until the first half of the nineteenth century that the significance of ciliated epithelium as a mechanism for cleaning the airways was correctly recognised by Purkinje and Valentin [350] and Sharpey in London [397]. At that time, mucous transit had already been observed by staining the mucus layer with dyes [24]. In 1877 Engelmann of Utrecht [112] demonstrated the 'ciliary mill': a strip of live ciliated epithelium was wrapped around a cylinder under gentle tension, producing rotation of the cylinder. Engelmann constructed an electric apparatus with contact points on the rotating cylinder at certain angles. The speed of rotation could thus be recorded without undue mechanical stress on the ciliary epithelium. He investigated the pharmacological effects on the ciliary epithelium by dripping substances on the preparation. A similar instrument – a cilioscribe – was designed in 1905 by Dixon and Inchley [90] and was also used for pharmacological investigations.

In the following decades of the twentieth century the physiology of ciliated epithelium was much investigated, notably by Antweiler [24], Dalhamn [80–82], Frenckner [130], Gray [146, 147], Herrmann [171], Hilding [178–186], Iravani [198–200], Lierle and Moore [238], Lucas [249–251], Messerklinger [278–288], Negus [303], Phillips [339], Proetz [343–345], Satir [394, 395], Swain [410], Tremble [437, 438] and Yates [474]. Much data was accumulated from experiments on animals and live human subjects about the mucociliary transport of the nose, the paranasal sinuses and the lower airways as well as the influence of temperature, humidity, ionising irradiation and many pharmacological agents.

Hilding [179] was singularly successful in demonstrating the energy of the ciliary epithelium. A decrease of pressure of 40 mm of water was produced in a hen's trachea connected to a U-tube manometer by the movements of an occluding plug of mucus. Hilding continuously propagated the importance of ciliary epithelium in the pathogenesis of many disorders, and encouraged clinical investigations. In 1960 he changed his designation from the 'slave-driver' of ciliary investigation to 'grandfather cilia' [186].

The development of the electron microscope provided a new impulse. Jakus and Hall [207] noted that the cilia of the paramecium contained longitudinal fibrillae, mostly 11 in number. Engström [113] in 1951 reported similar results about the cilia in the trachea of mammals. Detailed results of the electron microscopic structure of cilia were provided by Fawcett and Porter [120] in 1954.

The present investigation addresses the molecular mechanisms of the ciliary beat and its kinetic control, using electron microscopy, cytochemistry and intracellular potential recordings [83, 89, 254, 401].

3. Anatomy and Physiology of the Mucociliary System

3.1. Phylogenesis

The biological structure of cilia is phylogenetically very old. They are found in all animal species, even nematodes [400].

The ciliary structures serve several functions in their phylogenetic development. The paramecium possesses a continuous border on its under surface and this acts as a means of movement [303]. This ciliary function is very highly developed and probably lies under higher functional control, unlike the situation in man. Thus the paramecium can suddenly change the direction of the ciliary beat during flight [254]. A stream of water produced by cilia is used for digestion of food in mussels and oysters [303, 400]. In the frog, the palate and the entire oesophagus are lined by ciliary epithelium which provides an alternative to peristaltic muscle movement, and serves as a type of swallowing mechanism. In mulluscs and many fishes the exchange of water in the respiratory organs is sustained by cilia. Olfactory processes are also achieved by cilia, for example in the eel [303].

Cilia are found in the respiratory tract of vertebrates especially; they cleanse the walls in conjunction with the mucus. This mechanism is complemented by the cough reflex and the activity of the alveolar macrophages [372]. The movement of spermatozoa is also caused by a ciliary motor in the tail of the sperm. Thus the cilia are very important in reproduction, in addition to lining the fallopian tubes for the purpose of transit.

The ciliary structures have different functions, and thus have different names:

- Flagellae produce screw-like motions and thus a relative movement in the direction of the axis, for example in the sperm.
- Cilia produce a whip-like movement thus causing a relatively lateral movement, for example in the respiratory cilia, and in the movement of the paramecium [400].

Adjacent cilia, for example those in the respiratory epithelium, beat in time. However, since their movements are staggered in time, a continuous wave is produced like a waving corn field. This condition is termed metachrony, in contrast with synchrony. In a metachronous process there are three possible directions of the effective beat of the cilia, and thus of transit and the direction of the metachronous wave pattern:

– the effective beat and the metachronous wave run in one direction, termed symplectic metachrony.

– the effective beat and the metachronous wave run at 180°: that is antiplectic metachrony

– the effective beat and the metachronous wave run at 90° that is diaplectic metachrony which can be divided into laeoplectic which is directed to the left and dexioplectic metachrony which is directed to the right [400].

The various forms of metachrony are related to the function of the ciliary field. The symplectic type is unusual and is used for the purposes of movement in the opelina, a protozoon. The diaplectic type is used for the production of water streams, for example in the feeding processes of protozoa. The antiplectic type is the most common, and is found in the respiratory system of vertebrates [400, 401]. The length of the cilia is also adapted to their function. Thus cilia which move mucus are shorter than cilia which drive water [405].

During their further development the respiratory cilia probably lose the tactile sensitivity which causes resting cilia on the frog's palate to move in response to a mechanical stimulus. Also the neural control of the ciliary field which is present in the frog is lost in respiratory cilia [144]. Thus the ciliary motor in protozoa is capable of more differentiated action than the cilia of vertebrates [254].

3.2. Embryology

Cilia can be demonstrated in the human embryo from about the fourteenth week onward [68, 345]. It is not known whether they are capable of function at this time, since Ohashi and Nakai [313] found a functional maturation of the cilia of the trachea and nose of rabbits with respect to number, structure and direction of beat. It is thought that cilia undertake special functions during human development. Thus Afzelius [7] suspected that the visceral tube was rotated by the action of cilia. This observation is supported by the fact that molecular defects of the cilia in the immotile ciliary syndrome are associated with situs inversus in 50% of cases, suggesting random allocation. Svedbergh et al. [409] thought that the ciliary structures on the photoreceptors of the retina might align the receptors during development.

The speed of mucociliary transit during the first six months of postnatal development in lambs gradually approaches that of the adult animal, but the ciliary beat frequency remains the same from birth onwards [2]. The beat frequency is higher in the postnatal period in guinea pigs [27].

3.3. Site and Extent of Ciliary Epithelium in Man

It appears possible that almost every cell can form cilia [131] since each cell possesses the primary tubule apparatus in the form of a mitotic centriole which is also present in the cilium [7].

In the human, the nose, paranasal sinuses, nasopharynx, larynx and the lower airways as far as the terminal bronchioles are lined by ciliated epithelium [7, 198] with an estimated area of 0.5 m^2.

The eustachian tube and parts of the middle ear are also lined by ciliated epithelium [110, 300, 315, 384]. The number of cilia falls passing posteriorly from the opening of the eustachian tube into the middle ear. However the activity of the cilia increases the further they lie from the tubal ostium, and this might have a compensatory effect [316]. Felix et al. [122] could not confirm this finding in man. Whether the ciliary epithelium of the eustachian tube and middle ear is the most important factor in the cleansing mechanism, or whether the drop in pressure during swallowing is more important in transit, is yet undecided [106, 193, 417].

In the human genital tract ciliary epithelium is found in the efferent ductules of the epididymis, in the fallopian tube and neighbouring parts of the uterus [7]. It appears that a transit function is probable at both sites. The spermatozoa are driven forwards by a structure in their tails very similar to a respiratory cilium. Furthermore the ciliary epithelium is found in the ependymal lining of the ventricle of the brain, and it is suspected that it produces or complements circulation of the CSF [7]. Roth et al. [369] determined the ciliary beat frequency in preparations of animal ventricles. Structures resembling cilia are also found in the sensory organs. The cells of the olfactory epithelium bear cilia, but these are regarded as being immobile [7, 201]. Similar ultrastructures can be demonstrated in the inner ear in the kinocilium of the vestibule and of Corti's organ [7, 439]. Structures resembling cilia have been found in the retina and also in the epithelium of the internal surface of the cornea. It is suspected that they transport aqueous humour into the circular sinus of the iris close to the iridocorneal angle [409]. Cilia are also found occasionally in tissues where their function is very difficult to explain. Thus they are found in the brain, the pancreas, the liver, the kidney, the heart, connective tissue and the skin [7]. Ciliary epithelium has also been found in a cyst of the third ventricle, in an ovarian teratoma and in a parathyroid cyst [13, 335]. Cilia are often found in embryonic tissue, supporting the theory that cilia rotate the viscera [7].

The extent of ciliary epithelium in the airways is not constant, and appears to depend on environmental influences. The anterior third of the nasal respiratory epithelium can undergo metaplasia, due to exposure to the air stream [300]. Maurizi et al. [266] found ciliary epithelium extending to the vestibule of the nose in a nasal cavity which was not aerated, due to a unilateral choanal atresia, whereas metaplasia was found at the same site on the other side of the nose. They also demonstrated ciliary epithelium extending as far as the vestibule after laryngectomy [268]. Inflammatory conditions have a negative influence on the extent of the ciliary epithelium, for example in the nasopharynx [11].

Squamous metaplasia is often found in the subglottic space of adults whereas it is almost completely absent in the newborn [416]. Ciliary epithelium is typically found in the subglottis, in the ventricle and in other parts of the supraglottis which are less exposed to the air stream. Squamous epithelium is usually found on the vocal cords, on the opposing surfaces of the vestibular folds and in regions directly exposed to the air stream [47, 208, 414–416, 462]. At the anterior commissure there is a strip of ciliary epithelium joining the supra and subglottic spaces [51]. The epithelium of the posterior commissure is thrown into folds. Squamous epithelium is found on the tops of the folds, whereas ciliary epithelium is found in the depth [180, 437].

The extent of the ciliary epithelium in the airways is thus determined by environmental influences, such as the air stream, in addition to genetic factors.

3.4. Anatomy and Physiology of Cilia

Anatomical investigation of the component parts of a cilium was made possible by the development of the electron microscope [113, 120, 361, 362]. Current knowledge of the anatomy of the cilia will now be

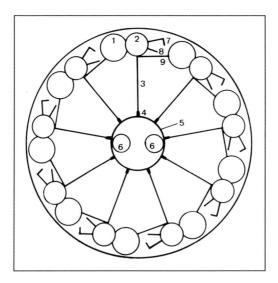

Fig. 1. Schematic cross-section of the ultrastructure of a cilium. 1: B microtubule, 2: A microtubule, 3: spoke, 4: spoke head, 5: central sheath, 6: central microtubule, 7: external dynein arm, 8: inner dynein arm, 9: nexin link.

summarised [9, 89, 254, 300, 401]. The cilia are protrusions of the cell membrane ensheathed by a double membrane. A ciliated epithelial cell carries between 50 and 300 cilia on its surface. In the era of light microscopy it was often stated that the number of cilia per cell was less [24, 281]. Reports of the ciliary mass vary between wide limits: the extent depends on function in the human, in animals and in protozoa. Thus, cilia which transport watery solutions are longer than those which move mucus. Also the cilia in the smaller airways in man are said to be shorter than those in the trachea and nose [341]. The length of mucus-transporting cilia in vertebrates is 3–8 μm; the diameter lies between 0.1 and 0.3 μm, with a narrowing towards the tip of the cilium.

The ciliary shaft contains nine peripheral double tubules and two central single tubles (see fig. 1).

The peripheral double tubules are arranged regularly and consist of two microtubules termed A and B. The double tubules are connected to each other by nexin links in such a way that they are mobile. Furthermore a connection is provided by an inner and outer dynein arm from an A microtubule to a B microtubule of another pair of tubules. Electron microscopy and biochemical studies [137] have shown that the dynein arms are morphological substrate ATP-splitting proteins, and thus can be regarded as the actual energy source of the cilia. Longitudinal preparations have shown that these dynein arms are present every 24 nm along the tubule.

The two central tubules are surrounded by their own sheath. Nine proteins extend radially from the peripheral tubules to the central sheath. These radial spokes are important for the stabilisation of cilia during movement. The spoke head, a thickening of the radial spoke as it approaches the central sheath, is also thought to consist of ATP enzyme splitting material [9]. The main direction of beat of the cilia is characterised by the position of the two central tubules; it lies perpendicular to the connection between the two tubules. The ciliary tubule has multiple connections to the overlying membrane along the entire shaft and especially at the tip of the cilia [89]. Small thorn-like structures are occasionally found on the cell membrane of the tip of the cilia, especially on the cilia which move mucus [89, 360]. These probably act like small claws to improve transit of the overlying mucus layer. Ring-shaped membranous structures are found close to the cell surface of the cilia bearing cells in the cell membrane of the ciliary neck which are known as the ciliary necklace. These are thought to be ion transit channels, especially for calcium [89, 254].

The root of a cilium lies within the cell, as a basal body, also termed the centriole or kinetosome. The two central tubules can no longer be demonstrated at the point of entrance into the cell, whereas the peripheral double tubules are continuous with the triplets in the basal body. Fibers are found on the cell body anchoring it to the cell membrane, and a rootlet extends within the cell. A spur or foot on the basal body indicates the direction of the effective beat.

Various theories have been developed to explain ciliary movement. Initially it was believed that the cilia were moved by repeated squeezing of cytoplasm like a hollow tube [117, 345]. Also the ciliary energy source was believed to lie in the basal bodies [361]. However current knowledge supports the theory of sliding filaments [5, 394]. The double tubules can move relative to each other with the help of the formation of alternating attachments of the dynein arms, like the actin-myosin mechanism in muscle movements (see fig. 2). Bending depends on fixation of the double tubules in the basal body, and on the structure-maintaining central elements of the ciliary axonems. The beat of the respiratory cilia resembles a whiplash.

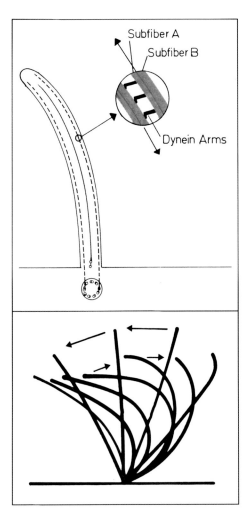

Fig. 2. Diagram of the mechanism of the sliding filament.

Fig. 3. Diagram of the ciliary beat.

The cilia are upright and rigid during the effective beat, whereas they are curved during the recovery phase (see fig. 3). Thus it appears that intermittent stiffness of the cilia is an important pre-requisiste for orderly function [154, 190]. Stiffness and active bending of the ciliary axonems alternate during the various phases of the orderly process of the beat at determined points on the axonem. Thus a co-ordinating mechanism must be present, but its nature is unclear. The ciliary beat is not produced exactly in one plane. The cilia deviate slightly laterally in the recovery phase so that the effective beat is not exactly linear. The tip of the cilia thus describe an ellipse [405]. It is suspected that ciliary activity depends on ATP: this would explain the marked collection of mitochondria close to the cell surface. The ciliary cells receive oxygen from the blood circulation and also by diffusion from the air present in the lumen. It appears that both sources of energy complement each other [97, 98, 358].

As already explained in the section on phylogenesis, ciliated epithelium is characterised by a metachronous beat. However, it is very probable that this process is not controlled by an intra- and inter-cellular coordination, but that it is a consequence of the close co-ordination with the overlying mucous layer as a mechanical necessity and ergonomic solution [254, 405]. The cilia beat with a frequency normally between 5 and 20 Hz, at 37 °C. However this rate is very dependent on temperature which must be taken into account: some authors do experiments at 30 °C and some at room temperature [79, 92, 95, 100, 115, 125, 228, 300, 334, 374, 377]. The frequency of the ciliary beat depends on the properties of the surrounding fluid medium: an increase in viscosity leads to a decrease in frequency [134, 198]. Frequency measurements during a period of several seconds subjected to fast Fourier transformation showed an apparently physiological variation of ciliary beat frequency of ± 3 Hz at temperatures above 30 °C [318]. This range was narrower at lower temperatures. The ciliary frequency in the tracheo-bronchial tree is not uniform and increases from the smaller to the larger airways. A physiological explanation would be the necessity for a higher transit capacity in the larger airways. The total extent of the smaller airways in relation to the extent of the trachea produces a more marked narrowing of the diameter available for mucus transit [198, 377], and this must be compensated for by increased transit capacity in the central airways. Similar concepts have been advanced for the nasal mucociliary transit [291]. Physiological regulation of the ciliary frequency of the respiratory epithelium of vertebrates has not been demonstrated, although neural control in frogs and various mussels is well known. Also local hormones such as serotonin can be demonstrated as the regulator in mussels [298]. In man the ciliary epithelium obviously works with an unchanging high activity [144, 400]. The pharmacological effect of the body's own substances will be considered in a separate section.

The origin of cilia from one cell is associated with the accumulation of an intra-cellular centriole on the apical cell membrane. From this arises the ciliary axonem leading to outgrowth of cilia from the cell. This process can be completed within hours [254]. The formation of cilia in respiratory epithelium is a continuous and ubiquitous process [15, 68, 131, 187, 281] which can be demonstrated dramatically by the scanning electron microscope [68].

This introductory section on ciliary physiology must of course be superficial and serves only as a basis for further discussion. Comprehensive monographs have been written by Sleigh [401] and Proctor and Andersen [341].

3.5. Physiology of Mucus

'The mucus is formed in the brain, it filters through the lamina cribosa and thus reaches the nasal cavity and then the outside'. Although Galen's concept [438] was refuted long ago, the exact origin and production of mucus in the respiratory epithelium surfaces still raises many questions. It has for a long time been known that 'drying is the greatest enemy of cilia', a fact which emphasises the importance of the mucus layer [345].

In 1934 the observation of active cilia in the presence of arrest of mucus transit led Lucas and Douglas [251] to propose that the mucus possessed a double layer. The cilia move freely in the sol layer close to the cells but contact only the undersurface of the gel layer; the effective beat thus produces mucociliary transport (see fig. 4).

The theory developed by earlier authors is still regarded as being valid. The concepts of arrest of the mucociliary transport, of 'empty' bearing cilia in a too thick sol layer, and of adhesion of cilia in a too thick gel layer were developed. Breuninger [50] was able to support this theory by showing that the mucus of the nose could change from an alkaline sol to an acid gel. Thus a pH gradient at the mucosal surface explains the double layer of the mucus. These two layers are visible on light microscopy, and could also be demonstrated by differential staining [4]. It is still disputed whether the gel and mucous layers are continuously present on the epithelium. Whereas earlier results cast doubt on this [199, 200], electron microscopy does indeed support the theory of continuity [35, 291]. It is possible that there are differences between the large and the small airways [341]. Also the concept of a relatively straight dividing surface between the sol and gel layer [384] has been brought into question by electron microscopy [360]. Thus the gel layer projects into the periciliary space. The mucosal gel originates from mucosal glands but the origin of the sol layer (also called the periciliary fluid) is still unknown. It arises either in the sero-mucinous

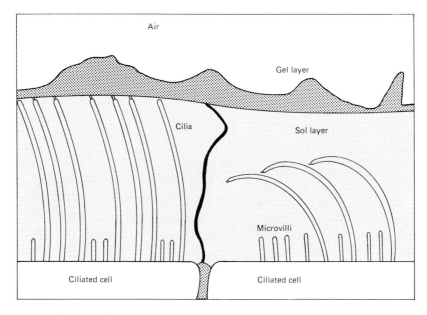

Fig. 4. Diagram of normal mucociliary transport.

glands [299] or by transudation and resorption directly through the cell membrane [337, 405, 431]. The presence of many microvilli between the cilia on the cell surface and the sub-epithelial fenestrated capillaries indicates a direct transudation through the cells achieved by an ion pump which draws its energy from the rich provision of mitochondria under the cell surface. Also the electrical potential found on the mucous surface supports the theory of an active ion transit [158, 466]. The air conditioning capacity of the nose should also be borne in mind: the correct mucosal layer necessary for mucociliary transport is maintained under various environmental temperatures and relative humidity. The nose can deliver up to 400 ml of fluid per day for humidification of the inspired air [340, 342].

Mucus consists of 98% of water, the rest being formed of albumin, globulin, glycoproteins and salts [384, 466]. In vivo, fibrous cords, the debris of cell membranes and small foreign bodies, are carried away in the mucous layer.

Harmsen et al. [165] found that the particles which reach the alveoli were probably initially phagocytosed by alveolar macrophages and then carried away with the cells in the mucus. The thickness of the mucous layer is very variable and lies between 0.5 and 10 μm [360].

Further investigations of mucus are faced with the problem of obtaining a specimen which is as natural as possible [105]. In animal experiments a large amount of mucus can be collected by creating a blind sac in the trachea. It can be mixed and preserved by deep-freezing, and later thawed again [140, 141, 384].

The mucus of respiratory epithelium is not only viscous, but also possesses elasticity due to molecular cross-linkage. The physical properties are thus described by two parameters, firstly the elasticity (storage modulus) and secondly viscosity (loss modulus) [73, 135, 140, 141, 162, 221, 258, 347, 384, 464]. Investigations of mucociliary transport using mucus of defined visco-elasticity have shown that a specific elasticity leads to optimal transit speed, whereas the influence of the viscosity is less important [245, 246, 355]. Also, the optimal elasticity can be demonstrated by changes of the cross-linkage of the mucus [135]. The mucus of different species is said to have similar functional capabilities [383]. Mucociliary transport can be produced by substances of the same visco-elasticity but different chemical composition, for example agarose, acryl amide gel, and gelatine gel: thus the physical properties seem more important than the biochemical.

Mucociliary transport requires an intact, metachronously beating, ciliary epithelium, and also an accurately balanced mucous layer of optimal visco-elasticity.

3.6. Normal Mucociliary Transport

The direction of mucociliary transport is normally the same in all humans [278, 438]. Similar conditions are also found in animals [40, 183, 251]. If a piece of mucosa is excised, turned through 180° and then re-implanted, the cilia retain their previous direction of beat. After mucosal injury the regenerating ciliary epithelium normally adapts itself to the direction of beat of the surrounding mucosa [345]. The controlling mechanism is unknown.

Mucociliary transport can be bridged at areas lacking ciliated epithelium by the traction exerted by the viscous mucous layer. This is known from the bridging of an incompletely re-epithelialised tracheal anastomosis [139] and from traction in a posterior direction on the metaplastic areas of the anterior parts of the nose [286]. Also a change of direction of the transit can be produced by the same mechanism by obstacles to the direction of beat. Hilding [184] demonstrated this phenomenon by transverse incisions in the mucosa of the trachea. Thus, a change in viscosity of the mucus could lead to a change of direction of the transit [284].

The direction of the mucociliary transport is independent of the position of the body. In 1924 Yates [474] showed by marking the mucus that the nasal transit was in a posterior direction towards the nasopharynx. Several authors have investigated the direction of nasal transit, both in animals and man [251, 278, 339, 341, 351, 399]. In animals, transit in an anterior direction from the superior turbinate is occasionally demonstrated [251], whereas in man an anterior mucociliary transport is only found at the very anterior end of the septum [341]. The transit is towards the nasopharynx in all other parts of the nose. Septal spurs or other obstacles are thus circumnavigated [138, 351]. The main streams meet in the choanae where a pathway leads laterally, on the posterior surface of the soft palate, to the lateral wall of the nasopharynx. Mucus carried to the posterior surface of the soft palate is then transferred to the posterior wall of the pharynx by movement of the soft palate [278]. The streams ending on the posterior edge of the septum then lead either to the roof of the nasopharynx or to the soft palate. A pathway from the lateral nasal wall passing above the opening of the eustachian tube leading into the nasopharynx has also been described [399]. Phillips [339] suggested in 1926 that nasal and sinus infections could often lead to otological diseases because the eustachian tube lies close to the main transit pathways (fig. 5).

Transport in the maxillary antrum follows a star shape, originating from the floor and ascending in a spiral to the ostium. Even after the creation of an antrostomy into the inferior meatus the stream of secretion is still directed toward the natural ostium (see fig. 6) [282]. The ethmoid and sphenoid sinuses empty directly into the ostium. Messerklinger's studies [283, 285] have shown specific transit pathways in the frontal sinuses. Two streams predominate: a lateral stream to the ostium from the lateral part of the floor of the frontal sinus, and a descending stream in the lateral part of the frontonasal duct. However an ascending stream can be demonstrated in the medial wall of the duct extending as far as the intersinus septum. Only a part of the mucus is drained into the nose from this circular traffic. If the viscosity of secretion is increased, this circular transport remains closed due to the traction phenomenon, leading to retention of

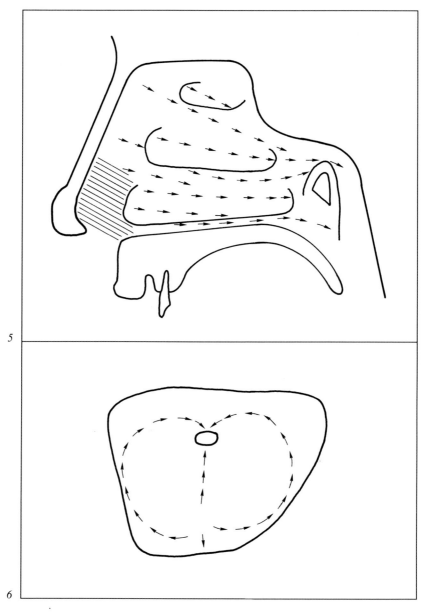

Fig. 5. Diagram of mucociliary transport pathways on the lateral nasal wall and in the nasopharynx. No transit occurs in the hatched area (see text).

Fig. 6. Diagrammatic view of the medial wall of the antral cavity with the maxillary ostium marked. The normal mucociliary transport directions are indicated by arrows.

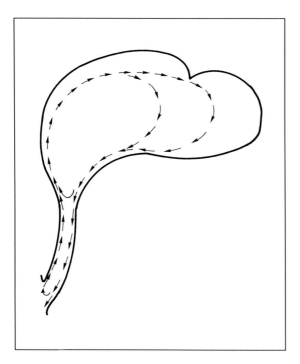

Fig. 7. Diagram of mucociliary transport pathways in a frontal sinus (modified from Messerklinger [283, 285]).

secretion in the frontal sinus. A small cell, the bulla frontalis (actually an ethmoid cell) can be identified which does not drain in accordance with this principle (see fig. 7).

The transit in the bronchial system is in an axial direction. At bifurcations the ciliary beat is so directed that secretions do not accumulate at a carina [198] (see fig. 8). There is some controversy about the transit pathways in the trachea, and some authors claim to have found an axially directed mainstream on the anterior and posterior walls [139, 182, 183, 199]. Other authors have found spiral [36, 303, 381] or zig-zag pathways [24]. However, all authors agreed that once this stream reaches the subglottis, all pathways are then directed posteriorly to reach the posterior commissure of the larynx [37, 51, 52, 118, 182–184]. It is said that there is a particularly rapid pathway on the posterior tracheal wall beginning at the bifurcation and ending at the larynx [471]. The streams arriving anteriorly at the larynx bend sharply posteriorly, when they reach the zone of transi-

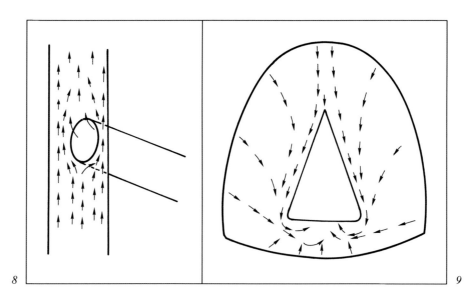

8   9

Fig. 8. Diagram of mucociliary pathways at the bifurcation of the bronchi.
Fig. 9. Diagram of a view into the subglottic space from the trachea. The normal direction of the mucociliary transport is marked with arrows.

tion to the squamous epithelium of the vocal cord, and then pass along the inferior edge of the vocal cord to reach the posterior commissure (see fig. 9). This pathway has also been shown by Zaitsu [478] in cats, and has also probably been confirmed by scanning electron microscopy. Normally the mucus is transported by the swallowing act from the posterior commissure into the hypopharynx [51]. Some authors have shown a transit pathway through the anterior commissure to the supraglottic area [39, 142].

Ardan and Kemp [25] suspect that movements of the larynx lead to contact between the vocal cord and vestibular folds, so that secretion which has accumulated on the inferior edge of the vocal cords is thus transferred to the supraglottic area.

Several investigations have demonstrated the phenomenon of whirlpools. These are small areas of rotatory mucociliary transport which form on folds and edges, and in the presence of increased viscosity of secretion. The secretion is clearly retained longer at such points [183, 199, 284].

The reduction in diameter of the intra-thoracic airways during expiration increases air speed and leads to friction on the mucosal surface which clears secretion [458].

4. Methods of Investigation of Ciliary Activity

4.1. Measurement of Ciliary Activity by the Reflex Method in vitro

In 1933 Lucas [250] first noticed that it was possible to observe the ciliary activity of respiratory epithelium under reflected light with relatively minor magnification. He used a beam of light kept cool by a heat filter and achieved a total magnification of 78 diameters. Further thinning for transmission microscopy was then unnecessary. Lucas was aware of the phenomenon of metachronous beat sequences and the formation of wave-like images. He considered that these waves explained the fact that the ciliary activity could be observed with lower magnification than was necessary for transmission microscopy. This method was much used in the following years [81, 130, 238] although the ciliary activity could only be estimated; alternatively the time course of the activity served as the measurable parameter [238].

Dalhamn and Rylander [80] were the first to carry out measurements with this method. They measured the changes in light by a photo cell with an appropriate amplification apparatus, and were thus able to measure the ciliary beat frequency. They demonstrated that such an apparatus was very sensitive to vibration [380]. In 1965 Hakansson and Toremalm [157] reported a technically refined method: the microscopic image was recorded by television camera and transmitted to a monitor screen producing a magnification of 1 in 10,000, whereas the actual optic magnification was only 40 times. The specimen was illuminated by a direct current light source screened by heat filters. The light changes are directly read off the screen with a small-surface photo-multiplier. The ciliary beat frequency was modulated to the frequency of the television screen and could be displayed and measured, using an electronic tube. This measuring system was soon adapted to newer electronic developments in signal processing [163]. However, the maximal frequency to be recorded was limited to 25 Hz by the television screen frequency. It is possible to record the average frequency every second and thus to illustrate the frequency over a long time, under varying experimental conditions [30, 134]. Similar measurements, but with an increased television screen frequency, were carried out by

Morgan et al. [291]. Chevance et al. [74], like Dalhamn and Rylander [80], used a cadmium photo-electric cell at magnifications between 40 and 80 diameters. Reimer et al. [354] used both the photo-multiplier and the photo-transistor, but preferred the latter because of the more favourable emission spectrum of the transistor and the unnecessarily high current of the photo-multiplier. Filtering of the initial signal from the light sensitive element is necessary for demonstration of the ciliary activity. Most authors achieve this with high and low pass filters which are strongly suppressive outside the band between 3 and 40 Hz [30, 195, 354]. The size of the light sensitive measuring spot on the mucosa is critical for good signal imaging, otherwise an average value is recorded of an excessive number of cilia which are not beating with a metachronous rhythm [74, 195]. Measuring surfaces 0.25 mm^2 in area [357], 100 micron in diameter [347] and 380 μm^2 in area [274] have been reported. Mercke et al. [274] achieved a signal-noise ratio of 24 dB with a photo-multiplier, a filter with marginal frequencies of 3 and 30 Hz, 100-fold magnification with the microscope and a measurement field of 380 μm^2.

It soon became obvious that the frequency and the amplitude of the signal vary [157]. Experiments into the cause of the light reflex change were set up by Toremalm et al. [428]. They measured the reflected light from a fluid surface stimulated by a tone generator and eliminated the formation of mucous waves by laying fine glass plates over the mucosa. Since a signal can be picked up from the mucosa by a glass plate, even if it is reduced in strength, they assume two sites of origin for the changes in light reflex:
1. Wave formations in the mucus.
2. Reflections at the ciliary apices in the mucus.

The variations of ciliary frequency make averaging over time necessary and valid. Intervals of 1 s [133], 20 s [197, 357] and 1 min [274] have been used. Puchelle et al. [347] carried out fast Fourier transformation of a signal interval and thus demonstrated the spectrum. It soon became obvious that the frequency measured on a mucosal preparation by the reflex method is not a measurement of the level of ciliary activity alone. The rheological properties of the medium overlying the mucosa determine the frequency, because increased viscosity of the medium reduces the frequency [73, 74, 134, 400]. Hybbinette and Mercke [195] reported their doubts about the local application of test substances to the mucosa, in the testing of pharmacological substances using the reflex method. Mercke et al. [274] demonstrated that two parameters are absent: the level of activity of the cilia themselves and the viscosity of the overlying medium.

Hakansson and Toremalm [160] noticed a signal change with a periodicity of 4–5 s in the wave sequences recorded from a tracheal preparation due to rhythmic contractions of smooth muscle in the tracheal wall.

4.2. Investigation of Ciliary Activity in vivo

The reflex method described above for the measurement of ciliary activity has also been used in vivo. Reimer et al. [355, 356, 358] opened the maxillary antrum of a rabbit from the lateral side and illuminated the mucosa of the opposite side of the antrum using an operating microscope so that the ciliary activity was made visible and quantifiable from the light reflex. The head of the anaesthetised rabbit was fixed in a rigid apparatus whose position could be adjusted with micrometer screws. Hybbinette and Mercke [195] and Mercke et al. [277] developed a model for pharmacological study on these same animals. They closed the fenestration with a heated glass window as previously described by Lierle and Moore [238] in 1935 and injected the test substances intraarterially [155]. Albertson et al. [17] used a similar method for a combined radiotherapeutic and pharmacological investigation. Reimer et al. [355, 356] used the reflex method with an operating microscope on patients undergoing a classical Caldwell Luc radical antrostomy. Normal ciliary activity was only recorded during apnea. The recording was distorted by the transmitted vibration of the cardiac action, respiratory activity and possibly muscle action, as could be recorded from the light reflected from an aluminium foil adherent to the forehead.

Toremalm et al. [429] found that the activity measured with the reflex method in vivo was higher than that in vitro, and suspected that this was associated with the optimal rheological characteristics of the mucus in vivo.

Messerklinger [287] reported that the ciliary activity could be observed from the light reflex during nasendoscopy with a rigid telescope if the objective was close enough to the mucosa. However, measurements were not accomplished by this method.

4.3. Measurement of Ciliary Activity by Stroboscopy

Stroboscopy was used as early as 1884 by Martius [261] during light microscopy of ciliary preparations. Movements observed could be demonstrated in slow motion with a flashlight from a rotating disk; alternatively the frequency of the movement could be measured during immobility. The latter method is now more often used [147, 249]: it became more popular during the 1950s due to the technical advance of electronically produced flash. It was thus no longer necessary to change the stroboscopic disks to alter the flash frequency. Furthermore satisfactory brightness was guaranteed despite a shortened illumination time. In recent years stroboscopy has therefore been used alone [115] or as the reference method [473].

However, at a symposium in 1956 doubt was cast upon the value of stroboscopy [33, 144, 380]. Stroboscopy usually shows zones of varying activity so that the entire preparation can never be brought to virtual immobility by the stroboscopic method. Stroboscopy must therefore be regarded as a psychosensorial method of measurement. Iravani [198] reported similar problems, but could produce a homogeneous frequency by cooling of the preparation, and thus carried out comparative measurements. Also observation of the preparation at flash frequencies below the fusion frequency of the human eye (18 Hz) is very tiring since a continuous image is not formed [33]. Chevance et al. [74] examined stroboscopy critically in a comparison of methods, and noted that accurate measurement was only possible if an individual cilium was observed. However, the problem would then remain that the cilia with an effective beat phase and a recovery phase of varying speeds would not conform to the optimal observation criteria of stroboscopy. Also the measurement of harmonic higher frequencies carried the possibility of error.

4.4. Measurement of Ciliary Activity by the Laser

Lee and Verdugo [233, 234] directed a reduced beam from a helium neon laser onto a specimen of ciliary epithelium in culture. The laser light was originally accurately defined in frequency and phase: it changed in accordance with the Doppler effect by reflection from the moving cilia. The light was converted by a photo-multiplier to an electric signal allowing the beat frequency of the cilia to be measured by electronic processing of the data. Metachrony of the ciliary beats could also be demonstrated. The measuring surface in this method was only 15 μm in diameter, corresponding to a ciliary population of 200–300 cilia. The validity of the method was checked by microscopic high speed photography. The advantage lay in the great accuracy of this method, although the sophisticated apparatus has deterred other groups. Verdugo et al. [450–452] later used the laser on a bigger field to observe a larger ciliary population submitted to pharmacological experiments. They demonstrated the spectrum of frequencies by a fast Fourier transformation. Measurements using the laser, for example by a fibreoptic catheter [424], have so far not been carried out in vivo.

4.5. High Speed Photography

The movement is recorded with high speed films during observation of the cilia either by transmission microscopy or by observation of the light reflected from the mucosa. Initial reports of this method were given by Gray [147] and Proetz [343]. After development of the film the beat frequency can be measured on the screen. This method thus became the most reliable for determination of ciliary activity, and was used as the reference method [233, 234]. Dalhamn [82], Iravani and Norris Melville [200], and Toremalm [427] relied on this method using an image frequency between 64 and 700 per second. The latter allowed an accurate analysis of the beat phase under appropriate magnification. Chevance et al. [74] also used high speed photography and emphasized the technically important details such as a heat filter in the illumination beam, as well as separation of the microscope and the camera to prevent transmission of vibration. They demonstrated that the method was usually carried out badly because of the high cost of the film. Also the development of the films and the counting were time-consuming. Rossman et al. [365, 367] reported the use of video recordings through the phase contrast microscope. Image sequences up to 60 per second could be achieved with a special video movement analysis system which then could be observed immediately on the monitor.

4.6. Recording of Intracellular Potential

The groups led by Hakansson and Toremalm [158, 159] succeeded in recording the intracellular potential of ciliated tracheal cells using a micro-electrode. Potential changes of the same order of magnitude as the ciliary beat frequency were recorded. The potential recorded at the tip of an intracellular electrode was 30–40 mV. They also recorded intracellular potential changes and the ciliary activity using the light reflex method simultaneously [236]. There was a difference between the recordings which increased with falling temperature in the culture medium: the frequency recorded by the reflex method was significantly lower and the intracellular frequency higher. The investigators found an effect of increasing viscosity of the mucus surrounding the cilia. This method did not demonstrate whether there is a frequency difference between the beating cilia and the resulting mucous wave or between the cilia and an assumed intracellular pacemaker. Thus a uniform, non-phase displacing potential was recorded, although electron microscopy showed that each cell carried up to 300 cilia which beat metachronously.

4.7. Cytological Observation of Viable Ciliary Cells and Measurement of the Ciliary Beat Frequency

In 1930 Hilding [178] observed viable ciliary epithelial cells obtained from the respiratory mucosa. He found rotating and vibrating cells or cell complexes. The activity of the ciliary epithelial cells was quantified by other authors by means of rotation [32, 33, 79, 95]. Ballenger et al. [33] showed that the ciliary movement could be assessed in this way, and also the ability of the entire piece of epithelium to perform work with co-ordinated metachronal activity which was then expressed as rotation. They described cell aggregates which did show ciliary activity but which apparently could not originate purposeful movement. Several authors [28, 125, 262, 281, 294, 448, 449] have observed cytological preparations of ciliated epithelial cells and estimated the activity in various grades, assessed signs of metaplasia [449] or observed functional or morphological signs of impending cell death after a certain time interval [262, 281].

In 1962 Dalhamn and Rylander [80] described a method of quantifying ciliary activity in such a preparation. The intensity of the observation beam was modulated by active cilia and this change was converted into a signal by a photo-electric cell; the frequency of the signal corresponded to the ciliary beat frequency. Chevance et al. [74] developed this method of micro-photo-oscillography further, using a photo-multiplier and an electric filter. This principle was later adopted by many authors who introduced several technical and methodological variations [1, 14, 38, 49, 59, 71, 92, 218, 228, 229, 247, 300, 310, 318, 364, 368, 374, 377, 446, 468, 473]. The cytological material was removed from the respiratory mucosa, either with sharp curettes [100, 334], or under the operating microscope [95] or with small nylon cytological brushes [69, 228, 473]. Moistening of the brushes with the culture medium to be used is said to increase the cell yield [374]. The use of local anaesthesia, the choice of an appropriate culture medium and the temperature of the culture medium will be discussed later in this monograph. The diameter of the measuring beam, and the size of the measurement surface in the plane of the preparation are as important for the accuracy of this method as they are for the reflex method. Asynchronous activity is sometimes recorded from a measuring surface covering several cells, leading to difficulties in evaluation. However, a small measuring surface can produce too little light to allow a signal to be distinguished from the noise of the electronic apparatus. Thus measuring surfaces were attained whose diameter was of the same order as that of the length of the cilia (5–6 μm) [92, 148, 218, 300, 452, 473].

The use of a photo-multiplier [74, 218, 228, 229, 300, 368, 377, 446, 473] or a photo transistor [92, 310] for the opto-electronic conversion appears to have no appreciable effect on the results. Many authors recommend preparing the electric signal with a low-pass filter with a marginal frequency of 30–40 Hz to eliminate the high frequency noise of the multiplier and possible power variations [74, 92, 228, 300, 310, 377, 446, 473]. Thus illumination with alternating current which is usually provided on most microscopes can be achieved with a filter of satisfactory selectivity.

The ciliary beat frequency is counted either on a storage oscilloscope, on paper strips of a recorder or automatically by a counter triggered by the signal. Since the curve does not have a uniform outline but includes intermediate waves and changes of amplitude, the method of counting and the trigger threshold affect the results [92]. Fast Fourier transformation of the signal [218, 368] clearly shows a preferred frequency by the presence of peaks in the spectrum, although these can fluctuate by several Hz within seconds so that assessment over a certain time is recommended. Since active cells beat with a varying frequency in cytological preparations, values averaged over 3–30 cells are given by many authors [100, 148, 228, 247, 334, 377, 473]. It has also been proposed that only those cells which are still fixed to the basement membrane should be chosen for measurement [57, 247, 367, 377]. Thus, resonance phenomena between the cilia and the cell body are said to be excluded: they can influence the frequency measured. The vital cytological methods described have been used by a few authors in recent years to make simultaneous assessments of the number of cells harvested [38, 69, 95, 228]: the cells are divided into squamous epithelial cells, and active or inactive ciliated cells; their proportions are measured [38, 247, 334]. Voss et al. [453] developed a nasal cytological method using light and electron microscopy which could be used for screening for dysplastic epithelial cells to detect malignancy.

5. Methods of Investigation of Mucociliary Transport

5.1. Marking Techniques

Mucociliary transport can be observed in vivo by following bubbles embedded in the mucous blanket [37]. Naturally the method can be improved by the use of marking substances. As early as 1830 Sharpey [397] used pulverised charcoal. Numerous other substances have been used, for example lamp black by Yates [474], and 4% indigo carmine by Phillips [339]. Messerklinger [284] and Urban [447] used Indian ink, or Chinese ink [282] whereas in the living subject they used Dermatolpulver. In order to find the smallest amount of marking substance, for example after nasal passage into the nasopharynx, Messerklinger [278] recommends a trypaflavine and brilliant dianil green which then can be observed as a fluorescent dye under high dilution during examination with ultraviolet light. Other substances used include coal dust, quartz powder, aerosol, lycopodium spores, particles of cork, aluminium powder, glass, steel or lead spheres [24], particles of mercury [383], aluminium discs [346], food dyes [388], poppy seeds [217], graphite powder [411], particles of metal [380] and edicol supra-orange dye [284].

Not every marking substance is suitable for observation of the mucociliary transit. Thus, Messerklinger [284] described how methylene blue dissolves in the entire mucous layer, forms a ring and is only transported after a delay. Frenckner [130] used black pieces of paper to avoid osmotic effects on the mucus. Antweiler [24] observed that many different marking substances produce relative drying at the point of application, due to the hydrophilic effect, and delay mucociliary transport. For the same reason Passali et al. [325–327] recommended plant charcoal, which is insoluble. Marking substances made of glass or metal are similarly inert. Stenfors et al. [417] attempted to imitate natural conditions as closely as possible. They instilled Evans blue with rat serum as a pseudo-effusion into the middle ear of rats to demonstrate the drainage of effusions via the Eustachian tube.

5.2. Saccharin Test

In 1973 Andersen et al. [21] described a new method of demonstrating mucociliary transport in the nose. They used equal amounts of food dye in solution of dyed sodium saccharinate. The crystals were cut to a size of approximately 1 mm^3 and introduced moist into the nose of the test subject. They were placed about 1 cm behind the anterior end of the inferior turbinate on the medial surface of the turbinate, that is at a depth of 5 cm in the nose measured from the nasal tip. The test subject was asked to swallow every 30 s, and to indicate immediately he appreciated a sweet saccharin taste in the throat so that the transit time could be determined. Measurement of the distance between the nasal tip and the posterior wall of the nasopharynx allowed the speed to be calculated. The arrival of the marking substance can also be checked by inspection after addition of dyes.

This method is very simple. It has been used later by many authors with variation of the technical details. The size of the crystals used has varied from a diameter of 0.5 mm up to a diameter of 3 mm with a weight of 14 mg [19, 20, 55, 152, 265, 322, 334, 387, 460, 477]. Even the latter size of particle has been shown to be transported: Stewart [418] was able to report that the mucociliary transport functioned up to a load of 20 mg/mm^2 without ill effects. Some authors recommend that the test should be carried out on the side of the nose which is more patent at that moment, to exclude the effect of the nasal cycle [55, 346]. Transit is obviously slower in the very congested side of the nose [96, 346]. Passali et al. [325] have shown that the results do not depend on the position of the head, whereas Pedersen et al. [334] showed that with increased accumulation of secretion in the nose the saccharin test is apparently influenced by gravity and appropriate position of the head. Andersen et al. [21] and Grossan [152] showed that it is better to ask the test subject to identify only a change in taste rather than the onset of a sweet taste, to make the test more valid. Double blind studies carried out by Yergin et al. [477] have shown that expectation can influence the test subject. However, before scoring a test as negative it must be confirmed that the subject can identify the substance as sweet [149]. The saccharin test has also been reported using powdered saccharin [346] or a 20 μl drop of a saccharin-indigo-carmine test solution [94, 100]. The latter has the advantage that it can be prepared in an isotonic and neutral solution. It is assumed that the saccharin dissolves in the entire mucous layer [55, 94, 322, 325, 346, 387], and thus demonstrates transit in the thin periciliary fluid and not in the viscous mucous layer bordering the lumen. This explains the results of an investigation in which saccharin together with a non-soluble marker was applied and the various transit times were recorded [96, 325]. Under these conditions the result of the saccharin test must depend on the physical condition of the mucous layer [387]. Andersen et al. [21] criticised their own method because it determined only the fastest transit in the nose since the apex of the transit front stimulates the taste sensation, whereas assessment of average transit times would be more valid from a physiological point of view. Passali et al. [325] observed circadian rhythms, transit being slower in the evening. Maurizi et al. [265] found longer transit times in children without catarrh. With increasing age the values approached those of the adult. Repeat investigations on the same and on succeeding days showed variation in the results, but the differences were not statistically significant [192, 346].

Normal values for the transit time through the nose from the point of application to appearance in the nasopharynx have been reported as follows:

Amabile et al. [19]	15 min
Brondeel et al. [55]	4–16 min $\pm$ 9.5 min
Duchateau et al. [100]	12–15 min
Ginzel and Illum [138]	5–20 min
Golhar [143]	5–20 min
Ohi et al. [322]	13.5 $\pm$ 1.1 min
Sakakura et al. [387]	10–15 min
Watanabe and Okuda [460]	6.5–23 min $\pm$ 4.2 min
Yergin et al. [477]	6–7 min

The following speeds have been reported by measurement of transit over a measured distance through the nose:

Andersen et al. [21]	4.6 mm/min
Holmberg et al. [65]	4.6–12.3 mm/min
Maurizi et al. [264]	5.6–6.0 mm/min

Various definitions have been proposed of the end point at which the test should be regarded as negative. Whereas Yergin et al. [477] end the test after 11 min, Greenstone et al. [149] wait for 60 min. Most authors accept a value of about 30 min. However before diagnosing mucus stasis Andersen [personal commun.] recommends ensuring that the marker has been applied deep enough, and on the ciliary epithelium. Despite this precaution Ginzel and Illum [138] recorded mucus stasis in 3% of normal subjects; they terminated the test after 30 min.

Elbrond and Larsen [106] used the saccharin test to demonstrate mucociliary transit in the Eustachian tube. They applied the marking substance through a perforation in the tympanic membrane into the anterior part of the middle ear cavity and recorded a transit time of about 32 min before the taste stimulus was reported.

5.3. Isotope Methods

As early as 1955 Albert and Amett [146] attempted to determine mucociliary clearance in the lung, using a radioactive tagged powder. This method was initially used for observation of incorporated radio-activity using single detectors with a slit collimator directed upon two end points of a tracheal segment of known length [139, 141]. A measure of the retention of radiosensitivity in the lung could also be obtained with a large surface collimator [64, 66]. The development of the gamma camera with an attachment for electronic analysis allowed the demonstration of an image, and the creation of time-activity curves in regions of interest [51, 52, 296, 475]. The cameras were provided with a shutter with a small aperture for demonstration of small areas (for example of the larynx or nose) to magnify the object, the so-called pinhole collimator [51, 351, 399]. Radioactive marking points were made at the root of the nose, the external auditory meatus, and on the chest at the level of the bifurcation so that the images obtained with the gamma camera could be better correlated with the actual anatomy, and to allow markers of length to be recorded on the camera image [21, 216, 296, 475].

The metastable gamma emitting isotope stage technetium-99 which is used for other isotope investigations has also been used as the radioactive marker. Camner et al. [64] used ^{18}F, and Patrick and Stirling [328] used barium sulphate-133. Simon et al. [399] measured an excessive radiation dose with technetium and chose ^{51}Cr instead. Connolly et al. [77] marked particles of varying sizes with different isotopes (^{99m}Tc, ^{125}I). The energy level emitted varies so that various markers can be distinguished after application. The radio-active exposure has been shown to be roughly equivalent to that of a chest radiograph [331]. It has been confirmed by Ahmed et al. [11] by serial investigation using X-ray opaque markers, that the mucociliary transport is stimulated by local application of radioactivity. This is explained by increased release of ATP from the mitochondria by acute disturbances of membrane permeability [30] which increase the ciliary beat frequency.

Technetium-99m, as a pure technetium pertechnetate solution, has been used only by McLean et al. [270] and Giordono et al. [139–141]. Other investigators couple the technetium to substances of predetermined quality and size; the rate of expulsion from the aerosol and the transit characteristics on the mucosal layer can influence the outcome.

The following table gives a review of the various substances used:

Group	Material	Size
Yeates et al. [475]	albumin microspheres	1.4 µm
Wolff and Muggenburg [471]	albumin macro-aggregates	6–30 µm
Quinlan et al. [351]	ion exchange resin	500 µm
Müller et al. [296]	sulphur colloid	2.8 µm
McLean et al. [270]	saline solution aerosol	2 µm
Pavia et al. [331]	polystyrene particles	5 µm
Waite et al. [455]	sulphur colloid	no data
Kärja et al. [212]	human serum albumin solution	no data
Kaya et al. [216]	ion exchange resin	304 µm
Sakakura et al. [386]	ion exchange resin	500 µm
Simon et al. [399]	ion exchange resin	10–50 µm
Puchelle et al. [346]	ion exchange resin	250–350 µm
Bridger and Proctor [51]	albumin microspheres	15–25 µm
Bridger and Proctor [52]	ion exchange resin	500 µm
Nuutinen et al. [305]	serum albumin solution	no data
Ahmed et al. [11]	albumin macro-aggregates	no data
Afzelius [6]	saline solution aerosol	6 µm
Andersen et al. [21]	ion exchange resin	500 µm
Connolly et al. [77]	ion exchange resin	3–180 µm
Camner et al. [66]	teflon particles	6 µm
Foster et al. [126]	sulphur colloid	4–5 µm
Ruehle et al. [371]	erythrocytes	7.5 µm
Griffith et al. [151]	DTPA	0.6 µm

For studies in which the marker substance must be inhaled into the bronchial tree the particle size is critical for the point of deposition: the smaller the particles (particularly under 10 µm) the further they penetrate into the periphery of the lung. Whereas only relatively heterodispersive aerosols are produced with pressure inhalers [296], the ultrasound and spinning disc methods produce an aerosol which is mainly monodispersive [66, 126, 330]. Relatively large particles are placed directly on the mucosa for the investigation of nasal transit [21, 55, 216, 346, 351, 386, 399]; alternatively a solution can be dropped into the nose [212, 213, 305]. In addition to the particle size the type of respiratory cycle is also important in the pattern of deposition in the tracheobronchial tree. A spirometer should be used to check these factors [296, 330, 475]. Furthermore the expired radionuclide can be collected again in the aerosol for radiation protection [296]. Also pre-existing disease of the lung and bronchi show characteristic nuclide deposition patterns which can be recorded by spirometry [296]. Using isotopes, Yeates et al. [475] reported a normal tracheal transit time of 3.4–4.6 mm/min in man. The following normal values have been reported for nasal mucociliary transport:

Andersen et al. [21]	5.8–7.3 mm/min
Brondeel et al. [55]	5.3 mm/min
Burgersdijk et al. [59]	4–13.5 mm/min
de Espana et al. [116]	5.3 ± 1.4 mm/min
Kärja et al. [212]	5.8–13.5 mm/min
Kaya et al. [216]	5.7 ± 2.2 mm/min
Quinian et al. [351]	7 mm/min
Sakakura et al. [386]	7.5 mm/min
Simon et al. [399]	3.6 mm/min

Nuutinen et al. [305] reported slower transit times in children. Wolff and Muggenburg [471] found a particularly rapid mucociliary transport pathway on the posterior wall of the dog's trachea, and Pavia et al. [330] reported rapid clearance of a radioactive depot in the central airways. Simon et al. [399] also suspected that the mucociliary transport was not equally effective in all parts of the nose. They were unable to record a continuous speed by following the particle through the nose. Quinlan et al. [351], too, found higher transit speeds in the posterior part of the nose. Using isotopes, Puchelle et al. [346] found marked daily differences in nasal clearance in the same subjects. It is also worth mentioning that Giordano et al. [141] described normal tracheal transit in dogs subjected to transverse resection and re-anastomosis of the trachea.

5.4. Radiological Methods

In 1956 Birzle [48] reported that the mucociliary transit could be followed radiologically in tracheal preparations using lead shavings, and he
investigated certain pharmacological and radiological questions. Bridger
and Proctor [52] demonstrated tracheal and laryngeal mucociliary transport by radio-opaque tantalum dust in animals. The radiological method
of demonstrating mucociliary transport is used more often in animal
experiments, and is also often used as a comparative method for isotope
investigations. Barium sulphate [328] and radio-opaque teflon discs [1, 11,
132, 382, 471] have also been used as markers. Friedman et al. [132]
developed the technique; they punched out pieces of teflon strip mixed
with bismuth 1 mm in diameter and 0.8 mm thick. These were then blown
through the channel of a fibre-optic bronchoscope into the trachea of the
experimental animal. Wanner [456, 457] used this method in man: the
introduced disks and then followed them by radiographs focussed on the
trachea at time intervals. Saketkhoo et al. [391] and Yergin et al. [477]
introduced radio-opaque teflon sheet into the nose and were then able to
demonstrate transit with repeated radiographs. Values for nasal transit
speed between 6.4 and 7.0 mm/min [471] and 6.6 and 9.4 mm/min [391]
were recorded. Radiological methods have not been widely adopted in
clinical practice, because of the risks of repeated exposure. A new approach
for determination of clearance of dust from the lung was reported by
Cohen et al. [76]: inhaled magnetite dust particles (Fe_3O_4) were aligned by
a strong external magnetic field. Once the magnetic field is turned off a
residual magnetic field can be measured which is proportional to the number of magnetite particles remaining in the lung. In this way, long-term
clearance investigations can be carried out without radiation exposure. It
is to be expected that this method will be developed further with techno-
logical improvements which allow imaging.

5.5. Endoscopy

Mucociliary transport can be observed by endoscopy. Transconioscopy, that is endoscopy of the subglottic space using a rigid endoscope introduced through the conus elasticus, was developed by Martensson et al.
[259]. This method allows mucociliary transport of mucus in the subglottic
space to be observed. The mucous transit can be followed easily by obser-

vation of air bubbles included in the mucous layer, or by introducing a dyed powder on the mucosa [118]. Bartholmé and Karduck [37] found that observation of mucous transit during transconioscopy produced diagnostic information.

Sackner et al. [381] described a method of observing the mucociliary transport in the trachea by fibre-optic endoscopy. Teflon slices 0.68 mm in diameter were blown through the working channel of a bronchoscope into the trachea. The transit of the particles was watched by endoscopy. The transit speed could be calculated by watching the course of these particles on film. Sackner et al. [381] carried out experiments on tracheal models and designed formulae for calculation of the transit speed. This method has been used on man: it is well tolerated and is practicable [392]. Mucociliary transport within the maxillary antrum has also been observed by endoscopy after marking of the mucus, and this technique is said to improve the diagnostic ability of endoscopy [43, 425]. Passali et al. [327] observed transit of carbon powder by the fibre-optic endoscope.

Ewert [117] developed a method of measuring mucociliary transport in man. The operating microscope was focussed on an area of the nasal septum in which the mucociliary transport proceeded at right angles to the axis of observation. The speed of the mucociliary transport could then be determined with a graduated eyepiece after marking of the mucus with a dye.

Important data about the mucociliary pathways in the nose and the nasal sinuses of the human cadaver were obtained by Messerklinger [283, 284, 286]. The mucociliary mechanism continues for up to 48 h after death, so that it is possible to inspect the nose and sinuses from an intracranial route after removal of the floor of the anterior cranial fossa. The transit of secretions can thus be studied after marking of the mucus.

5.6. Discussion of the Method of Animal Experiments

Engelmann [112] used the frog's oesophagus which is lined with ciliated epithelium for driving the ciliary mill. Later the frog's palate was frequently used as the model for mucociliary investigations. Giordano et al. [140] demonstrated that the rheological results obtained were applicable to studies on the mammalian trachea, whereas Lucas and Douglas [251] and Messerklinger [281] emphasised that the ciliated epithelium of the frog's palate is normally at rest and only becomes active after mechanical stimulation. Thus the validity of this model is doubtful, since other regulatory mechanisms are obviously at work. Pharmacological and rheological investigations have been carried out mainly on fresh preparations from animals which had been sacrificed [24, 182]. The dog's trachea [140, 373, 398], the dog's frontal sinus [339], the paranasal sinuses and trachea of rats [251, 328], the nose of cats [24, 251] as well as those of mice and rabbits [251] were used. Iravani [198] developed a method in which the intrapulmonary airways of the rat were freed from the surrounding lung tissue under the microscope. The ciliary beat and the mucous transit could be studied through the intact wall of the bronchi and bronchioles. Ukai et al. [443, 444] used the hen's antral cavity, a structure that can be inspected easily through the mouth. Humanoid apes are the closest animal model to man, but require a great deal of care and are very expensive [467]. It remains to be mentioned that basic investigations of cilia are carried out on protozoa or molluscs [254, 401].

6. Culture Methods

6.1. Culture Methods for Cytological Investigation of Viable Material

Particular demands are placed on the culture medium used for cytological experiments to maintain the viability of cilia bearing cells. It is naturally important whether representative measurements can be taken within the first hour or whether the action of drugs can be observed in vitro for up to 24 or even 48 h.

The hanging drop [79, 181, 229], or a concave or cylindrically ground slide with a cover slip, are used for short term investigations [473]. For longer investigations the Rose or Dvorak-Stotler chambers are used. This apparatus is formed of several layers and air-tight chambers screwed together. It possesses a small channel through which the culture medium can be renewed or changed for controlled pharmacological experiments [33, 79, 176, 229, 452]. In longer experiments it is important to prevent drying of the preparation by sealing [79].

Dolowitz and Dougherty [91], unlike Ohashi and Nakai [310], found that a simple saline solution was insufficient for a culture medium since morphological disorders of the cilia and cells occurred. Therefore, they used Locke-Ringer solution, but achieved the best culture results with the patient's own serum. All authors have shown that it is important to pay attention to the physiological osmolarity and the pH [79, 100, 176, 376]. Various ready-made nutrient media are available as the basic medium. They include Gey's, Eagle's, Liebovitz's, Hank's and Earl's solutions [79, 95, 102, 150, 176, 377, 473]. Special buffer systems such as Hepes or Tris buffer, or other additives such as glutamine, hydrocortisone, pigs' insulin, fetal calves' serum, ampicillin, penicillin or streptomycin, are often added. It is claimed that the length of physiological culture can thus be prolonged. However, Tris buffer has a very unfavourable effect on ciliary activity [348], as does deficiency of the calcium ion [451].

6.2. Culture of Mucosal Preparations

Certain conditions must be fulfilled to allow observation of ciliated epithelium of a mucosal explant for several hours. Hilding [181] described a specially constructed box in which he could transport the mucosal transplants and protect them from cooling and drying. Special chambers have been described [217, 276, 347, 354] in which measurements could be undertaken at constant humidity and temperature. The mucociliary activity can be recorded using the reflex method through a window protected against condensation by a special heater. Humidified test gases can be introduced into this chamber for experimental purposes. The ciliary activity remains viable for several days using such methods [262]. Drying of the mucosa produces paralysis of the mucociliary activity, probably due to increased viscosity which can be prevented by a sol spray [283]. Proetz [343] constructed a special small irrigation-suction apparatus for mucosal preparations. If mucosa is observed in vivo, the animal's fluid balance must be maintained [195, 380]. Iravani [198] reported a special preparation technique for the observation of the intrapulmonary airway in fluid.

If a mucosal preparation is cooled, normal mucociliary activity is resumed when it is warmed again [48, 282]. Thus under some circumstances the survival of the preparation can be prolonged for several days after death. After considerable efforts, Hilding [182] found that storage of the preparation at room temperature in a closed plastic bag did not appreciably restrict its usefulness.

6.3. Long-Term Culture of Ciliated Epithelium

Long-term culture of ciliary epithelium in which cell division occurred was achieved for the first time in 1936 by Proetz and Pfingsten [344]. Ciliated epithelium was taken in utero from the nose of guinea pigs, and was successfully cultured in a solution consisting of culture medium and the mother's serum. Growth was observed from the second day onwards. Dedifferentiation or overgrowth by fibroblasts did occur, but ciliary beat could be observed all over the new epithelial surface. Proetz followed the dynamics of the cell culture with fast motion film.

Hoorn and Tyrell [194] also carried out cultures over several weeks. Ballenger et al. [33] showed that dedifferentiation of the cells can be prevented by accurately estimated supplements of vitamin A. Also an increased ambient CO_2 content produced a larger proportion of active cells [99]. Burkert [62] reported cell cultures of human adenoids which could be grown for several weeks. The ciliary beat under the influence of various pharmacological agents was observed using a photometric method. Ohashi et al. [321] also reported long-term culture of ciliary epithelium.

7. Microscopic Methods of Investigation

7.1. Light Microscopy

Light microscopy is frequently used in simple morphological investigations. Numerous detailed descriptions of ciliated epithelium and its normal constituent cells, such as ciliary and non-ciliary bearing cells, goblet cells and basal cells, have been given [98, 300, 434]. The proportion of leukocytes in the epithelium and the stroma has been determined in disease [205, 469]. Based on the height of the epithelium and the content of the secretion of the goblet cells, Messerklinger [279, 280] showed that the ciliated epithelium has a functional cycle under the influence of the autonomic system. Metaplasia and degeneration of the epithelium as a reaction to external stress has also been well recorded by light microscopy [60, 185]. Zilliacus [479] in 1905 described a dye method for macroscopic differentiation of squamous and ciliated epithelium of the respiratory tract: the respiratory epithelium was stained red and the squamous epithelium yellow. Doubts were cast on the validity of this method because of artifacts due to autolysis [208]. Stell et al. [414–416] described other macroscopic staining methods and checked the validity by histological serial sections.

Light microscopy has recently been expanded by histochemistry and autoradiography [467]. Thus the epithelial cells can be investigated thoroughly by immunohistochemistry for the presence of primary filaments [337]. Determination of enzymes by histochemistry provides information about the functional condition [262, 295] and the proliferation can be assessed by autoradiography of the synthesis rate of RNA [262].

7.2. Methods of Taking and Processing Ciliated Epithelium for Electron Microscopy

It is not the purpose of this article to illustrate the current methods of transmission and scanning electron microscopy whose significance in research in the ciliary mucosa is already well-known [203]. However, brief comment will be made on the demands on time and personnel, and on the considerable manual skill required for successful electron microscopy.

Rapid fixation of the specimen is important since autolysis can very rapidly change the ultrastructural appearances. Reissig et al. [360] irrigated viable ciliated epithelium with the fixation solution under the preparation microscope. Morgan et al. [291] fixed the animal preparation by intravascular perfusion, and by the injection of formalin vapour into the trachea. Kotin et al. [230] instilled fixation solution into the trachea. Rautiainen et al. [353] found that glutaraldehyde and cacodylate buffer are optimal; artifacts were possibly due to brisk shaking.

The principal danger during preparation of the mucosa is that the surface is covered by mucus so that the ciliated epithelium itself remains concealed. Lenz [236] and Werner and Privara [462] rinsed the specimen in physiological saline and succeeded in washing off the mucous layer. Naturally this procedure precludes immediate fixation. Stretching the piece of mucosa on a surface facilitates orientation and finding of the ciliary blanket [465], and prevents contraction of the specimen leading to the appearance of folds on the surface [271]. Hilding and Hilding [187] first looked for ciliary bearing areas using light microscopy, and then embedded the areas of interest for ultra-thin sections. Of the various fixation methods only that reported by Fox et al. [128] will be mentioned: it is claimed that the addition of magnesium ensures better demonstration of the dynein arms.

Viable human specimens for electron microscopy are most easily obtained from the nose, but the specimen must be taken from a sufficient depth to ensure that cilia are found [173]. Sufficient cellular material can be obtained without local anaesthesia using a cytological brush, thus preventing pharmacological artifacts [68, 149, 264, 374]. A specimen can be taken from the nose with a small forceps with [128] or without [337, 469] local anaesthesia, or using a sharp ring curette [367]. Bryan et al. [57] prepared electron microscopic specimens from mucous smears. The thinnest sections possible are necessary to demonstrate the ultrastructure of the cilia well in cross-section. Fox et al. [128] demonstrated the value of tilting the specimen through several degrees during microscopy to compensate for minimal oblique incision. Takasaka et al. [422] photographed cilia under the electron microscope and prepared a composite view of nine exposures by rotating the ciliary cross section through 40° between exposures. In this way an averaged virtual image of the peripheral double tubules could be demonstrated. Afzelius et al. [10] even succeeded in making longitudinal measurements of sections of cilia.

Electron microscopic pictures are increasingly being submitted to morphometric analysis to provide quantifiable results [68, 69, 291, 378, 467]. Counting of electron microscopic ciliary anomalies per number of cells must be regarded as a further improvement: Mygind et al. [301] did this on coded preparations to eliminate observer error.

8. Morphological Changes in Ciliated Epithelium

8.1. Metaplasia

About 80% of normal epithelium in the airways consist of ciliary cells, the remainder being goblet cells [236, 311]. The structure of the epithelial layer is not entirely uniform throughout the entire respiratory tract. The cells in the paranasal sinuses are rather cuboidal whereas they are more columnar in the well aerated parts of the nose [345]. Increased exposure to air leads to epithelial metaplasia [203]: squamous metaplasia is found anteriorly where the vestibular squamous epithelium gives way to respiratory epithelium in the normally aerated nose. This area cannot be demonstrated in the affected side of the nose of patients with choanal atresia, indicating the causal relationship with exposure to air [266]. In the larynx, squamous epithelium is found mainly in those parts exposed to the airstream [47, 415]. Scott [396] found squamous metaplasia on the free edges of the vestibular fold; its frequency and extent increased with decreasing distance between the free edges of the vestibular folds. This finding supports the conclusion that metaplasia is mediated by increased mechanical stress. Metaplasia of the respiratory epithelium is seen more frequently in the larynx of older subjects [47, 396], whereas in the newborn only the vocal cords are covered by squamous epithelium [416].

In chronic inflammatory lesions of the respiratory epithelium the proportion of goblet to ciliated cells increases until eventually only occasional ciliary tufts can be demonstrated by scanning electron microscopy [311, 356]. Clear ciliary cells with swollen cytoplasm are found, and the number of cilia per cell falls. More free leukocytes are found in the epithelium and entire epithelial cells are lost. Ohashi and Nakai [311] observed ultrastructural changes in the ciliary cells indicating direct transformation into goblet cells; a sharp increase of the rough endoplasmatic reticulum was also seen. It is not known whether these cell transformations take place directly, or whether they are due to metaplastic regeneration after damage to the basal cell layer [60]. Other signs of early metaplasia include increased number of axonemata in a sheath, and the formation of intracellular tonofilaments [311] as well as desmosomes [360]. Typically, superficially damaged and metaplastic ciliated epithelium shows an increased number of microvilli strewn over the cell membrane of the superficial undifferentiated cells [110, 164, 236, 311, 449].

The reaction pattern of ciliated epithelium to an inflammatory stimulus appears to be entirely monomorphic, with loss of cilia and ciliary cells in favour of goblet and undifferentiated cells [236, 311, 356, 449]. Damage due to ionising radiation leads to atrophy of the entire epithelium, with reduction in the number of goblet cells [18, 85, 110, 370]. Squamous metaplasia can be produced experimentally by deprivation of vitamin A [360]. Mechanical damage, for example due to prolonged intubation, causes cell loss extending as far as the basal cell layer [363].

The intact ciliary blanket, even if it is no longer capable of function, protects from microbial invasion [103].

8.2. Acute Desquamative Lesions

Ciliary cells undergo extensive acute desquamation during a common cold [172, 178]. This desquamation appears to be a typical result of viral infection, whereas bacterial inflammation leads to protracted cell damage. Exacerbation of this reaction pattern occurs in allergic airway disorders, and in pulmonary infection with mycoplasma [7].

Papanicolaou [323] termed the desquamation ciliocytophoria. Only about 10% of the surface is covered by ciliary epithelium in the acute phase of the common cold [469], and only a few ciliary cells can be demonstrated in cytological smears taken during a common cold [334].

Acute desquamation can be produced experimentally by various different gases [60, 467]. Ultrastructure shows a coalescence of the mitochondria and a loosening of the intercellular connections leading to cell loss. However, loss of the cilia is not inevitably associated with death of the entire cell [467].

8.3. Regeneration of Ciliated Epithelium

The dramatic loss of ciliary epithelium in a common cold inevitably raises the question of the mechanism of regeneration. It is generally accepted that the ciliary epithelium regenerates from the remaining basal cell layer [47, 345, 362, 419, 467]. Regeneration from the margin of the damaged area is often limited because of the extent of the lesion. Also doubt is often cast on the transformation of mature goblet cells to ciliated cells and vice versa [47, 362]. Rapid cover of the epithelial lesion is first achieved by an acute metaplastic regeneration [60], arising from poorly differentiated cells, so-called intermediate cells, capable of differentiation in various directions [467]. Continuing stress leads to differentiated squamous epithelium [47] whereas withdrawal of noxious influences leads again to the formation of ciliary epithelium [60]. The regenerated ciliary cells are said to carry fewer cilia initially than normal [35]. After operations on the nasal sinuses or the nasopharynx the layer of ciliated epithelium reforms provided that marked submucosal scarring has not been caused by the operation [303, 345]. Also a continuous layer of respiratory epithelium is developed after a tracheal anastamosis, and this can resume full transit function [139]. The regenerated ciliary carpet in the paranasal sinuses resumes mucociliary transport in the same direction as before [345].

The time taken for regeneration varies, and the type and extent of damage obviously needs to be taken into account. The cytology of the nose returns to normal about 14 days after a common cold [334]. Ewert [117] also could no longer find squamous epithelium at exposed points in the nose 14 days after laryngectomy. Metaplastic regeneration occurs within three weeks of tracheal anastomosis but is only converted to a complete layer of ciliary epithelium six months later [139]. After chemical injury [60] the epithelium regenerates in 8–10 weeks. Rhodin [362] found evidence of a constant change in respiratory epithelial cells. Carson et al. [68] were able to confirm this with electron microscopy and also found evidence of constant ciliogenesis in the cells. Tos [435] suspected that the cell cycle of ciliary epithelial cells lasts about 14 days.

8.4. Ultrastructural Pathology of the Cilia

Many disorders of the ultrastructure of cilia are now well known, thanks to scanning and transmission electron microscopy.

The typical arrangement of microtubules in the ciliary shaft with nine peripheral double tubules and two central single tubules can be abnormal. Thus additional peripheral double or single tubules may be found, so that the axonem normally described by the term 9 + 2, is then described as 10 + 2, 11 + 2 or 12 + 2. Peripheral tubules may also be deficient. Disorders of the numbers of the central tubules are often combined with a deficient number of peripheral tubules (9 + 0, 8 + 0), or superfluous peripheral tubules (9 + 4, 10 + 4). A finding of deficient central tubules must be interpreted with caution since the central tubules end close to the surface of the cell and are also difficult to demonstrate at the tip. A transverse section with a 9 + 0 structure is thus also possible with a normal cilium [7, 8, 21, 13, 119, 129, 174, 175, 205, 264, 367, 388, 422, 455]. A transposition of tubules, that is a central displacement of peripheral double tubules, is also found. However, this anomaly can be demonstrated only if the appropriate area of a cilium is cut in longitudinal sections [78, 175, 290, 367, 420].

The direction of ciliary beat is determined by the position of the central tubules, and is at right angles to the connection between the central pair. If a group of cilia is found in cross-section under the electron microscope the direction of the beat can thus be determined. Rautiainen et al. [352] have provided a statistical method for calculating this. Normally the direction of beat should have a maximal divergence of 26° [174]. A higher divergence, or random arrangement of the direction of beat, is pathological. An increased number of these abnormal findings must be assessed critically since twisting or change of position of cilia can occur at a greater distance from the surface of the cell, and this can conceal disorientation. The direction of the effective beat can also be deduced from the spur on the basal body [7]. If a superficial section reaches this area it is a reliable indication of the orientation of the beat.

Often several normal or abnormal axonemata are found in a cytoplasmic protrusion. These structures are termed giant cilia, megacilia or compound cilia; they can contain as many as 40 axonemata. Giant cilia which are slender and without any appreciable cytoplasmic excess (adhesive type) can be distinguished from a sac-like type with larger cytoplasmic protrusions (bulging type) [422]. Mecklenburg et al. [271] observed cilia which had coalesced like a brush at their tips; they were regarded as the preliminary stage of a giant cilium of adhesive type [13, 15, 114, 119, 129, 131, 174, 175, 205, 264, 311, 367, 426, 433, 465, 470]. A doubling of the basal bodies was described by Burian and Stockinger [61]. Occasionally axonemata were also found which were clearly intracellular. This finding is usually interpreted as a disorder of ciliogenesis [8, 15, 61, 175, 433]. Afzelius et al. [10] found abnormally long cilia and concluded that this indicated disordered transit function. Physical insults such as heat or ionising radiation produced nodules on the ciliary shaft visible on scanning electron microscopy. Under the transmission electron microscope they appeared as vesicles and possibly cytoplasmic protrusions [17, 31, 131, 264, 271, 311, 462].

Bertrand and Degen [42] found kinks of the ciliary shaft at the tip, and termed these hockey stick cilia. Swellings were also found on the ciliary tip [264]. An important finding was reported in the middle 1970s by Pedersen and Rebbe [332] and Afzelius [6]. They found a deficiency of the dynein arms which normally unite the peripheral double tubules and which are regarded as the ATP splitting proteins, the actual energy source. This deficiency of external dynein arms has been later confirmed by many authors in specific diseases [12, 72, 78, 123, 125, 150, 174, 175, 205, 213, 264, 426, 449, 455, 460, 465].

The inner dynein arms are technically difficult to demonstrate so that the finding of a deficiency of inner arms requires validitation of the method [149, 301, 334]. Watanabe and Okuda [460] suspected that the dynein arms could not find the correct binding point on the opposite tubule, and this could produce motility disorders. Sturgess et al. [420] found cilia in which the radial spokes connecting the peripheral tubule with the central structure as well as the central sheath could not be demonstrated. This produced a decentering of the central tubule which was said to influence the stability of the cilia especially during bending. A cleft of the peripheral tubule pair has also been described [367]. Infection with mycoplasma is said to produce a specific disorder of the ciliary necklace where important ion channels can be observed [8].

These numerous descriptions prompt the question as to how far such disorders of structure produce disorders of function [174, 264]. Biochemical investigations show that the defect of dynein arms as an ATPase protein leads to disorder and loss of function [137]. Also the number of dynein arms present and the area of the arms in cross section correlate with function [378]. It might be suspected that a giant cilium with 30 axonemata does not function normally, but this is difficult to demonstrate. Rossman et al. [366] found typical movement patterns in certain specific ultrastructural defects. The ultrastructural defects were mainly found in patients with demonstrably abnormal mucociliary function, supporting the conclusions about the functional relevance of ultrastructural pathology. On the other hand, it cannot be refuted with certainty that morphological anomalies may be due to the chronic inflammatory change in the mucosa.

Ciliary anomalies are not necessarily found on all cilia demonstrated. The significance of ultrastructural investigations is greatly increased by quantification of the anomalies relative to the total number of cilia [69, 124, 129, 203, 367, 455, 470]. It is so far unknown what incidence of abnormal cilia causes disorder of the entire mucociliary transport system. Estimates begin at a proportion of 40–50% of the population [72, 264]. It must also be remembered that 3–5% of cilia are atypical in apparently healthy subjects [69, 470].

The difficulty of recognition of structural details under the electron microscope at the necessary magnifications raises the question of failure in the method. Mygind et al. [300, 301] carried out investigations with coded preparations, and found overlap and lack of definition between clinically clearly distinct cases. These sources of inaccuracy are naturally greatest in assessment of the smallest structures such as the dynein arms and radial spokes. There are also often problems in finding sufficient, exactly transverse, ciliary sections [59].

Ultrastructural disorders are divided into genetically determined and acquired ones [8]. Defects in the dynein arms and radial spokes, as well as tubule transposition, are genetically determined, since they are often found not only in respiratory epithelium but also for example in the tail of the sperm of the same individual. Furthermore these disorders are usually found only in diseases manifest since birth [69, 214, 470].

The remaining ultrastructural changes are found both in acquired and experimentally produced circumstances. It is accepted that acquired ciliary anomalies are produced by physical or chemical injury or by chronic inflammation. Giant cilia, intracytoplasmatic cilia and numerical aberrations of the configuration of the tubules are thought to be associated with disordered ciliogenesis. Furthermore, in genetic ciliary disorders, in addition to the typical ultrastructure, other lesions are described which are probably caused by inflammatory changes associated with primary disordered mucociliary transport [109, 205].

9. Pathophysiology and Pharmacology of the Mucociliary System

9.1. Pathology and Therapeutic Influence on the Mucous Layer

The problem of the pathology of the mucous layer of the respiratory epithelium lies mainly in the method. Animal experiments with creation of a tracheal pouch for the collection of mucus showed that a specific viscoelasticity produces an optimal mucociliary transit. In the human, it is difficult to collect bronchial or nasal mucus in which the normal physical and chemical properties are preserved. The method of intratracheal viscosimetry described by Kuschnir [231] requires a tracheostomy. An alternative method of collection from the nose [105] is mainly indicated for biochemical and chemical investigations. The expectorated sputum cannot be regarded as representative of the mucous layer which produces the mucociliary transport since a healthy subject usually cannot cough out secretions [372].

There remain investigations of the method relating to the entire clearance of the respiratory epithelium, and whose results have not yet been discussed. Whether increased or reduced clearance is produced by an effect on the mucosal layer or on the cilia remains largely unanswered [312]. Experiments have shown that changes in viscosity produced by various mucolytic agents alter mucociliary transport [67, 260, 284]. An increase of the ciliary beat frequency in response to mucolytics has also been observed experimentally. However a change in viscosity of the periciliary fluid level can produce this effect without a change in rhythm of the ciliary pacemaker [155, 200].

Andersen and Proctor [22] suggest that not every mucolytic agent improves mucociliary transport. It is known from clinical experience that coughing, the second bronchial clearing mechanism, can be improved by mucolytics and by increased secretion. Brown et al. [56] reported mucolytic treatment of secretory otitis media, and mentioned that the clearance of the middle ear was mainly based on functioning mucociliary transport, since the pressure changes due to tubal movements were an ineffective analogue of the cough reflex.

Before considering the effect of pharmacological agents on the mucociliary system the physicochemical conditions for mucociliary function must be discussed.

9.2. Physicochemical Conditions

The first physiological investigations of ciliary activity by Engelmann [112] in 1877, as well as those by Dixon and Inchley [90] in 1905 were concerned with the temperature dependence of ciliary activity. Engelmann found increasing activity up to 45 °C followed by rapid decline. The optimal ciliary beat frequency thus lay between 30 and 40 °C, but mainly in the range of the normal body temperature [62, 198, 218, 228, 310, 345]. The temperature limit above which ciliary stasis sets in has been reported by different authors to lie at 40 °C [310], 42 °C [198], 43 °C [345], 51 °C [275] and even as high as 55 °C [218]. The lower limit for ciliary stasis has been reported as being 4–7 °C [198, 303], but the cilia are reactivated on rewarming.

Proetz's [345] dictum is often quoted: 'The only natural enemy to cilia is excessive drying.' Proetz observed a localised ciliary disorder under a fine airstream directed on the mucosa. The optimal relative humidity is said to be around 90%. Mercke [276] and Toremalm et al. [429] showed that at higher temperatures the mucosa reacts with a decrease in activity to reduction of relative humidity.

Quinlan et al. [351] observed a reduction in the nasal mucociliary transport when they maintained the relative humidity of the inspired air at less than 30%. Systemic dehydration to a tolerable degree does not lead to inhibition [140]. The ciliary activity is optimal at a pH value within the neutral range [217, 252, 345]. pH values between 7 and 10 are tolerated without any appreciable effect, whereas ciliary stasis rapidly set in outside these values [92]. In the mucosal unit, pH values of between 2 and 9 are tolerated without reduction of transit.

Correct osmolarity is necessary for normal activity, as was discovered long ago by Engelmann [112]. Hyper- or hypo-osmolar solutions rapidly led to loss of activity [62, 92, 303, 345]. Ciliary function depends on a satisfactory oxygen supply to the cells [97], although only small amounts of oxygen suffice [430]. The supply of oxygen can be maintained at normal levels, not only by diffusion from the circulating blood, but also by diffusion from the surface [358].

The effect of ionising radiation has been investigated several times; it has great therapeutic importance [17, 30, 85, 169, 289, 315, 345]. All investigators have found an increased activity in the first phases of irradiation which is explained by increased ATP accumulation due to disorders of membrane permeability. Increasing doses of irradiation lead to disordered function, and eventually to irreversible immobility.

Ultraviolet light also is said to inhibit mucociliary transport [48]. A certain mechanical load on the mucociliary epithelium, for example by blood clot or mucus, produces acceleration [198].

9.3. Pharmacology of the Mucociliary System

Investigation of the pharmacology of the function of the mucociliary system presents problems of methodology. The various techniques of pharmacological investigation include the following:

1. Individual ciliary cells in culture are treated with the test substance, and changes in beat frequency are measured. This is a demanding method for the observation of single effects on the cilia.
2. An excised strip of mucosa is kept in culture and treated with the test substance. The beat frequency of the mucociliary epithelium is determined by the light reflected from the metachronous waves. The presence of a mucous layer is important since changes in viscosity can influence the beat frequency.
3. In the animal, an area of mucosa can be demonstrated in vivo and the beat frequency determined by the reflex method. Test substances can be applied locally or systemically. Possible changes in viscosity of the mucous layer must be allowed for.
4. A test subject or an experimental animal is exposed to a test substance, either locally or systemically, over a longer period. The ciliary beat frequency is then determined in vitro from a viable cytological smear. In this method complex interactions such as dilution, changes in the test substance and pharmacokinetic effects must all be taken into consideration.
5. An isolated piece of mucosa is exposed to the test substance, and the speed of the mucociliary transit is measured.
6. The test subject or an experimental animal is exposed to the test substance, and changes of mucociliary transit are measured in vivo by various methods.

It should be noted that methods 1-4 mainly determine the ciliary component whereas methods 5-6 assess the entire transit capability including the effect on the mucous layer. In the in vivo investigation using method 4, and method 6 especially, the other pharmacological effects of the test substance which can lead to secondary effects on the parameter measured must also be assessed. For example it has already been mentioned that mucociliary transit in a non-congested nose is quicker, a fact which is important in the testing of nasal drops. In bronchopulmonary investigations, bronchial constriction or dilation must be taken into account in the method. For this reason the same or similar drugs can produce apparently contradictory results which can be explained by differing methods of investigation.

9.3.1. Physiological Regulators, Biogenic Amines and Transmitters

Fundamental pharmacological investigations have been carried out in a search for substances which can regulate ciliary activity by physiological means. Thus Gosselin [144] found that serotonin affected the cilia of mussels, and he thus regarded this substance as a regulator hormone. However Hybbinette and Mercke [195] observed no effect due to serotonin in mammals, even in sublethal doses. Histamine, gamma-aminobutyric acid [144], vaso-active intestinal peptide, encephalin [242] and calcitonin-gene related peptide [277] could not be demonstrated to have an effect on the cilia. On the other hand nasal mucociliary transport was reduced by the application of histamine in man, but this was possibly determined by altered mucous secretion or by swelling [447].

Prostaglandin E_1, E_2 and $F_{2\alpha}$ were found to stimulate ciliary activity [200, 450]. ATP and other triphosphorylated nucleotides stimulate cilia in vitro, and this was prevented by AMP and ADP by receptor blockade [209]. ATP has no effect on mucosal preparations in vitro [195], whereas the nasal mucociliary transport is said to be accelerated by local application of ATP solution [306-308].

Investigations with transmitter substances have been carried out in a search for a suspected physiological regulation of mucociliary activity in the nose and paranasal sinuses. Acceleration of transport was induced by mechanical stimulation in the hen but could be prevented by prior administration of parasympathicolytic drugs [444].

Extensive investigations have been carried out by Mercke's and Lindberg's group [195, 239-243, 277]. Substance P which is excreted in response to stimulation of the C fibers of the maxillary nerve leads to

Table 1. Accelerating effect of sympatheticomimetic substances

Adrenaline [195]
Orceprenaline [195]
Isoprenaline [197, 229, 248]
Isoproterenol [452]
Terbutaline [229, 312]
Reproterol [176]
Salbutamol [197]

ciliary acceleration. Substance P could be demonstrated by immunohistology in the maxillary nerve, the sphenopalatine ganglion and submucous nerve bundles. Acceleration was also produced by capsaicin, neurokinin A and bradykinin, but each of these was blocked by an antagonist of substance P, emphasising the importance of this transmitter. Lindberg et al. [243] suspected the presence of a mucociliary protective reflex which is activated by ammonia vapour or exposure to cigarette smoke.

9.3.2. Sympathicomimetic and Sympathicolytic Agents

In earlier experiments 1:1000 epinephrine applied to the epithelium had an inhibitory effect [238, 345]. More recent investigations with other concentrations of sympathicomimetic drugs have shown stimulation of ciliary function (see table 1).

Clenbuterol could not be shown to have any effect on ciliary function [155]. Alpha-sympathicomimetic drugs inhibit cilia [195, 197] an action probably mediated by beta-receptors. This is supported by investigations with specific receptor blocking substances which have no effect but which prevent stimulation produced by mimetics [197, 229, 248, 452]. Beta$_2$-mimetics are unanimously regarded as important agents.

Also the entire mucociliary transport was accelerated by sympathicomimetics in in vivo experiments [66, 121, 227, 229]. However, on occasion no such effects [67, 331, 385], or only brief effects [336] were found.

An increased transit capability produced by terbutaline, but only in patients with bronchitis [392], favours the proposal that improved mucociliary clearance is a secondary effect due to improved aeration produced by bronchodilatation. The effects due to sympathicolytic agents such as propanolol [331] and reserpine [442] were variable.

9.3.3. Parasympathicomimetic and Parasympathicolytic Agents

Parasympathicomimetic substances such as acetylcholine, metacholine, pilocarpine [195, 196] and carbachol [49] had a stimulating effect on ciliary function in vitro which could be blocked by parasympathicolytic agents which on their own had no effect. However, ciliary beat frequency decreased in cytological smears in vitro [71]. Ipratropium bromide led to a doubtful ciliary stimulation [14, 229].

Atropine slowed tracheal mucociliary transport [24, 140, 475], whereas the cholinergic agent bethanecol had an accelerating effect [331]. Ipratropium bromide in the bronchi and nose showed no specific effect on mucociliary transport.

9.3.4. Local Anaesthetics

The local anaesthetic agents used on the mucosa such as lignocaine, cocaine, procaine, dibucaine and tetracaine all show a dose-dependent reduction of ciliary movement [79, 294, 303, 345, 374, 376, 445]; they may even produce immediate ciliary paralysis. However Rutland et al. [376] showed that there was no significant difference in beat frequency in vivo in response to 4% lignocaine, in comparison with the untreated side of the nose. Objections to the clinical use of this local anaesthetic are thus not valid. Mostow et al. [294] showed additive ciliotoxic effects due to the stabiliser substance methyl-hydroxy-benzoate (Methylparaben).

9.3.5. Mucolytic Agents

Mucolytic substances such as calcium iodide, bromhexine, and guaifeninsin increase bronchial clearance, whereas N-acetylcysteine, S-carboxymethylcysteine and ambroxol produce varying results [67, 260, 331, 461]. Bromhexine and its metabolites have not been shown to affect ciliary activity.

9.3.6. Other Agents

It is generally agreed that theophylline and aminophylline improve mucociliary clearance from the bronchi [229, 331, 408]. Naturally, the bronchodilator effect must be taken into account in assessment of the method. Penicillin produces abnormal mucociliary function, whereas gentamycin has no effect [345, 430].

Provocation of the respiratory tract by allergens reduces the transit capability, but this can be prevented by the prior administration of sodium chromoglycate [457].

Direct application of alcohol in high concentration to ciliary epithelium leads to disordered activity [48, 235, 345].

Misonidazole used as a radiosensitiser potentiates the radiation induced reduction of ciliary beat frequency [17].

9.3.7. Nose Drops

Decongestant nose drops are sympathicomimetic substances which have been shown to inhibit cilia [432]. Only Saketkhoo et al. [391] have been able to demonstrate accelerated transit in vivo in man using phenylephrine and tetrahydrosoline. Other authors [94, 399] have observed retardation. The injurious effects on the ciliary epithelium of stabiliser substances such as benzalconium chloride, chlorbutol, thiomersal and EDTA have been investigated in vitro [93] and in vivo [94].

Topical glucocorticoids such as budesonide and betamethasone do not damage the transit or the ciliary function in vivo; they inhibit the cilia when used in vitro [101, 382, 413], and produce transit disorders after prolonged use [192].

9.3.8. Cigarette Smoke

Contrary to expectation, nicotine applied to an in vitro preparation initially causes an increase of ciliary activity and then reduction of ciliary activity several hours later [32]. The action of the whole smoke on such preparations is harmful [181], and the smoke of non-filtered cigarettes has even more marked effects [81, 82].

The action of cigarette smoke on the mucociliary transport is inhibitory, both in vitro and in vivo, and differences can be found between filter and non-filter cigarettes [67, 217, 327]. The pure nasal mucociliary transport is similar in both smokers and non-smokers [351, 399]; only one group has found a different result [327].

9.3.9. Anaesthesia

The significance of temperature and relative humidity for the function of the mucociliary system is discussed in Section 9.2. The fact that the oxygen supply of the mucociliary epithelium can be provided via the blood circulation and also via the luminal air is also discussed at that point.

Ciliary function is optimal at an atmospheric oxygen concentration of 20%, although disorders do not occur even at a concentration of only 1% in a nitrogen atmosphere. Pure oxygen has no ciliotoxic effect [430]. The tolerance interval to anoxia is about 20 min [358], although morphological changes can be demonstrated within 15 min. Bronchial clearance may even be accelerated at a 50% oxygen content [151].

There is controversy about the effect of pure nitrogen and carbon dioxide [358, 430]; ciliary inhibition may occur at a carbon dioxide concentration of 5 kPa [359].

Tracheal transit is slowed in response to ether and chloroform [48]. Proetz [345] was able to produce immediate ciliary paralysis by the administration of drops of ether, whereas an ether atmosphere had no demonstrable effect on a mucosal preparation. He made similar observations for chloroform. Halothane reduces ciliary transit [70, 328], but nitrogen dioxide does not damage ciliary function, even in overdoses [345].

Thiopentone and pentobarbital slow tracheal transit [328, 381] whereas morphine, fentanyl and sufentanil have no demonstrable effect [170]. A faster mucociliary transport is observed in response to high frequency oscillation of nasal air at frequencies between 8 and 20 Hz [136].

The effect of high frequency respiration on marginal particles was investigated by Gruenauer and Grotberg [153]. The views of Warwick [458] on the varying diameter of the airway in inspiration and expiration should be consulted. It is also worth mentioning that the effect of high frequency respiration on the rheological properties of bronchial mucus are controversial [156].

9.3.10. Industrial Exposure

Since the ciliary epithelium comes into close contact with pollutants in the environmental air, numerous investigations of industrial exposure have been carried out.

Sulphur dioxide is an important element of industrial air pollution. In several investigations it has caused reduced mucociliary clearance [1, 22, 442]; the threshold for damage lies between 1 and 5 ppm. Also combinations with ozone [1] and plastic dust [22] showed harmful effects. Ozone alone in a concentration of 0.2 to 0.4 ppm [127] accelerated tracheobronchial clearance [127]. An aerosol of sulphuric acid reduced clearance [244].

Formalin vapour and solutions below 0.25 ppm inhibit ciliary movement [167, 217, 292], and also disturb nasal transit [34].

Disorders of nasal clearance have been demonstrated in a cohort of woodworkers [20], and damage to ciliary movement has been found after prolonged exposure to chromates [262]. Andersen [22] gives a comprehensive review of the industrial medical aspects of the mucociliary system.

10. Specific Syndromes

10.1. The Immotile Cilia Syndrome: Primary Ciliary Dyskinesia

In 1966 Hilding [186] suggested that there was an entity of ciliary insufficiency. Pedersen and Rebbe [332] in 1975 discovered that ciliary immotility was caused by failure of the dynein arms. This finding was confirmed by Afzelius [6] who described the symptoms of infection of the upper and lower airway with possible situs inversus and male infertility. This group coined the term 'immotile cilia syndrome' [108].

Kartagener's syndrome consisting of situs inversus, nasal polypi and bronchiectasis is regarded as a partial expression of this new entity [7].

Sturgess et al. [290, 420, 421] found a defect of the radial spokes and a tubule transposition as further ultrastructural features of this syndrome, and distinguished three sub-types. Further investigation shows that mobile and ultrastructurally normal cilia can also be present in the immotile cilia syndrome [173, 448]. Rossman et al. [365, 366] and Rutland and Cole [375] described atypical movement patterns in patients and coined the term 'primary ciliary dyskinesia' which is now accepted by many authors [403].

The phenomenon of normal ultrastructure in patients with this syndrome was solved by a quantitative microscopic investigation [300, 333, 367]; this showed a distinctly higher proportion of the three typical ultrastructural anomalies in comparison with healthy subjects.

The incidence of the immotile cilia syndrome, or primary ciliary dyskinesia, varies between 1 in 15,000 and 1 in 30,000 [123, 150, 301]. Familial occurrence has been described, and it is suspected that the condition is an autosomal recessive hereditary disease [114] in which ultrastructural defects are not confirmed in other members of the family [104]. The frequency is increased in geographical areas with an increased proportion of intermarriage [8]. Functional and morphological primary cilia dyskinesia is found in Polynesian patients with bronchiectasis, and the high regional incidence is probably due to inbreeding [455].

Chronic infections of the upper and lower airway are characteristic of primary ciliary dyskinesia. Typically they are present from birth, and cause persistent catarrh [7, 39, 301, 324]: bronchiectasis frequently develops [366]. Chronic, usually secretory, middle ear inflammation can be observed also [72, 78, 114, 150, 204, 333, 366, 465]. However the rate of acute middle ear inflammations and the incidence of the common cold is said not to be increased [301]. The frontal sinuses are often described as being poorly pneumatised [7, 301], and polyposis does not typically arise in the nose and nasal sinuses [150]. According to the theory that cilia determine embryonal rotation, 50% of the subjects demonstrate situs inversus [7]. The full syndrome includes immotility of the spermatozoa, causing sterility. Female patients are said not to be inevitably infertile, and ectopic pregnancy is said not to be frequent as might be suspected in view of the provision of cilia in the uterine tube [7].

In a patient with typical symptoms the most simple specific diagnostic test [459] is the saccharin test described by Andersen et al. [21]. Investigations of the mucociliary transport in the bronchi and trachea are also seminal [8, 297]. Further steps would consist of cytological investigation of viable ciliary cells; the investigations should be carried out at various time intervals, especially in the absence of infection, to confirm the diagnosis [300]. A period which is as free as possible of infection should also be chosen for electron microscopy to avoid secondary ultrastructural changes [301, 326].

The diagnosis is not simple, because of the difficulties of quantitative electron microscopy [301], and because other conditions such as mucoviscidosis or immune defects associated with disease of the respiratory system must be distinguished. In addition to the costly electron microscopy, semiquantitative functional assessment of viable cytological smears is also widely propagated [28, 364].

Diagnostic criteria include the following [8]:
1. Chronic bronchitis and rhinitis.
2. Situs inversus occurring in at least one member of the family.
3. Viable but immotile spermatozoa.
4. Markedly reduced tracheal clearance speed.
5. Typical ultrastructural defects.

The contribution of early diagnosis to treatment is emphasised [63, 301] allowing timely introduction of physiotherapy for the lungs. Activation of immotile cilia by ATP and ATPase might open up new therapeutic prospects [125, 307]. Bronchodilators, mucolytic agents and antibiotics are recommended for pulmonary symptoms [125, 150, 431]. There is controversy about the place of surgical drainage procedures in the treatment of sinusitis. Some authors regard turbinectomy and intranasal antrostomy as a logical procedure for retention of secretion in the nasal sinuses [150] but it is also said that radical operations on the sinuses have not produced any long-term improvement [174]. However, others commend the results of surgery [114, 301]. The introduction of drainage tubes is universally recommended for the treatment of chronic middle ear effusions [114, 150, 172]. Toremalm [431] advises protecting patients with primary ciliary dyskinesia from ciliotoxic pharmacological agents and occupational exposure to injurious dusts or gases. Satisfactory humidification and abstinence from smoking are also recommended.

Patients with primary ciliary dyskinesia observed over a long period, do not suffer dramatic life-threatening deterioration of lung function, if care is good [78]. The pulmonary system is decisive for the vital functions; it is provided with the effective supplementary clearing mechanism of coughing.

10.2. Chronic Sinusitis

Messerklinger [282] found damage to ciliary function only in granulomatous mucosal sinusitis, whereas normal ciliary function was found in polypoid sinusitis. Normal ciliary function may be found even in an antral empyema [430]. Some have found no cytological evidence of reduced ciliary activity [149, 356, 367], others recognised inhibition of activity parallel with increasing metaplasia [310, 311, 319].

Disordered ciliary function is found in about one third of patients with chronic infection of the upper airway [59]. The ciliary action obviously cannot achieve normal mucociliary transport because of the altered visco-elastic properties of the mucus, as investigations of transit have shown [143, 145, 149, 206, 256, 264, 282, 305, 387]. Electron microscopy shows increased mucosal metaplasia in chronic sinusitis [15, 124, 311, 356] and in addition numerous aberrations of the tubules, vesicles in the ciliary shaft and frequent giant cilia. Defects in the dynein arms and radial spokes probably indicate a genetic defect [264]. Completely normal ultrastructure has also been found in sinusitis [149]. Ciliary ultrastructural changes are found in mycotic sinusitis [412].

Shortening of the disease process and increased activity of the mucociliary system can be achieved by terbutaline [311]. Alternatively the clearance function can be improved by conservative treatment [389]. The mucociliary transport is also optimised by operations to improve ventilation [138].

In immune defects the disordered transit can be improved by appropriate substitution treatment [214]. Adenoidectomy in children has been shown to restore mucociliary transport to normal, so that the saccharin test is recommended as a further method for assessing the indications for this procedure [267].

Reference to investigations of the action of micro-organisms on the mucociliary system is appropriate at this point. Bacterial infection is more likely in the presence of abnormal mucociliary function, as shown experimentally in the 1960s [35]. The effect of bacteria on the ciliary apparatus has been investigated thoroughly in the last few years. The effect of *Pseudomonas aeruginosa* or its metabolites reduces beat frequency [189, 357, 432, 468]. It is suspected that the mechanism is a membrane damage due to a protease [189] or a mitochondrial damage [357]. Ciliary disorders were demonstrated in response to *Haemophilus influenzae* [210, 468], *Diplococcus pneumoniae* [432], *Klebsiella pneumoniae* [320, 321] and leukocyte elastase [348], whereas staphylococci [219, 468], hemolytic streptococcus [432] and *Escherichia coli* [357, 432] showed no such effect.

10.3. Allergic and Vasomotor Rhinopathy

An allergic rhinopathy slows mucociliary transport due to altered composition of the mucus [26, 143, 216, 264, 446, 457]. Normal findings have been recorded in allergic subjects outside the pollen season [399]. A reduction of ciliary activity was observed during exposure to allergen in vitro [430]; others were unable to reproduce this effect [148] and ciliary activity has been observed reduced in allergic subjects [317]. It might be suspected that the initial lesion in allergic rhinitis does not lie on the cilium, and that the ultrastructural lesions are secondary in nature [111, 129, 264, 422]. Similar findings are recorded for vasomotor rhinopathy [129, 216, 236].

10.4. Common Cold

As early as 1930, Hilding [178] suspected that there was a disorder of mucociliary transport during a common cold due especially to injury to the ciliary component. Sakakura et al. [386, 443] confirmed the damaged clearance function in experimental virus infection, and found ultrastructural evidence of increased destruction of the ciliary apparatus [388]. Pathological electron microscopic findings of the cilia have been reported [69, 469].

10.5. Rhinopathy after Laryngectomy

A running nose is common in the first weeks after laryngectomy due to an excess of fluid, because of absent evaporation following loss of ventilation. It is remarkable that normal or even improved mucociliary nasal transit can be demonstrated after laryngectomy. This is explained by reduced exposure of the nasal mucosa to the environment [117, 216, 268, 281, 341, 351, 387, 399, 411].

10.6. Ear Diseases

Ear diseases have already been mentioned in the discussion of primary ciliary dyskinesia. These patients suffer from increased middle ear effusions [72, 114, 204, 301]. There is controversy about the importance of an intact mucociliary transport system in the eustachian tube for the normal function of the middle ear [193, 417]. The pathogenetic course is difficult to reconstruct since changes in the mucous component [56, 188, 269, 384, 423] and also disorders in the tubal mechanics [416] are decisive; furthermore primary and secondary lesions are very difficult to distinguish from each other. A correlation has been found between the transit function of the tube and the results of tympanoplasty [106]. Disordered mucociliary transport was marked in patients with cholesteatoma [45]. In secretory otitis media bacterial colonisation and the increased carbon dioxide partial pressure [359] were mentioned as the cause of the ciliary disorder [320]. There may be a correlation between the recurrence rate of the effusion and ciliary activity [454].

10.7. Mucoviscidosis

Mucoviscidosis is primarily a disease of the mucous component of mucociliary function. In vitro the ultrastructure and ciliary activity are normal [367]. Typically the tracheal clearance speed is markedly reduced [456]. The cilia demonstrate a kink at the tip which might be attributed to the thickened and highly viscous mucous blanket [161]. The serum of patients with mucoviscidosis has no effect in vitro on the ciliary activity of ciliary epithelium, disproving the existence of a serum-bound ciliary inhibitory factor [379].

10.8. Disorders of the Lung and Bronchi

The tracheal clearance speed is significantly reduced in 60% of young smokers [456]. The pulmonary clearance is also affected in chronic and allergic bronchitis [456, 457], although the bronchial ciliary activity lies in the normal range [228]. No significant abnormality of ciliary activity was found in patients with bronchial carcinoma [228], whereas ultrastructural evidence of a higher proportion of giant cilia has been reported [13]. On the other hand the mucociliary clearance was significantly reduced in patients with bronchial carcinoma, even in comparison with patients with chronic bronchitis [263]. Electron microscopic findings are normal in tuberculosis [12].

10.9. Eye Diseases

Corneal abnormalities are more frequent in patients with the immotile cilia syndrome, but have no clinical significance [407]. Since cilia could be demonstrated in the epithelium on the posterior surface of the cornea a causal correlation was suspected. On the other hand an increase in pathological ciliary ultrastructure has been found in the nasal epithelium of patients with retinitis pigmentosa [128]. There is speculation about the correlation with the inner ear deafness in retinitis pigmentosa (Usher's syndrome), since ciliary structures take part in the genesis of both these sensory epithelia.

11. Personal Investigations

Experience must first be gained with the methods described in the literature for investigation of the ciliary epithelium, to evaluate their place in the investigation of laryngeal carcinoma.

The nasal mucosa is very suitable for physiological studies of ciliary epithelium since it is readily accessible without causing undue stress for the subject. On the other hand, the ciliary epithelium of the larynx and the upper trachea is quite difficult to reach. Investigations of this area are relatively invasive and even dangerous, or must be carried out under anaesthesia. However, the latter method is unsuitable for physiological investigations since the effects of the anaesthetic agents must be taken into account.

The epithelia of the upper and lower respiratory tracts are very similar in their anatomy. They also react with remarkable similarity to diseases, for example, virus infections and allergy. Therefore it appears justifiable to use the nose as the model for the investigation of ciliary epithelium. Thus the preliminary investigations of the method used in this thesis were mainly carried out on the nasal epithelium.

11.1. Intravital Observation of the Ciliated Epithelium

The ciliary epithelium in the paranasal sinuses of patients was observed using the method described by Messerklinger [287] during endoscopy of the sinuses through the anterior wall of the antrum. Local anaesthesia was only used outside the antrum, thus eliminating a direct pharmacological effect on the ciliary epithelium. An opiate, a neuroleptic and atropine were used as systemic pre-medication. After making a stab incision in the canine fossa a trocar was used to perforate the anterior wall of the antrum. The mucosa was then observed using a rigid Hopkin's telescope after sucking out mucus or pus. A flickering movement representing the mucociliary wave pattern could be observed at the edge of the reflected light as the telescope approached the mucosal surface. Occasionally passing mucus could be detected by movement of an entrapped air bubble. This ciliary activity was found in antral cavities filled with mucus or pus. Also an antral cavity irradiated many years ago showed clear ciliary activity.

Quantitative assessment of ciliary activity using a method analogous to the light reflex method did not appear reasonable for methodological reasons. High magnifications must be used, as on the operating microscope, to allow measurement of the light changes with a phototransistor or a photomultiplier. These cannot be achieved with the normal endoscope. Secondary magnification by a further lens system is a possible solution, but it is likely that the vibration of the investigator's hand, as well as the respiratory movements and heart beats of both the patient and the investigator are an increasing source of error, which has previously been reported during intravital investigations, even under anaesthesia with an operating microscope mounted on a stand.

Repeated opportunities were available for observing ciliary epithelium in vivo during investigations or operations on the ear under the operating microscope. The mucociliary activity could be observed from the resulting light reflex, especially in the often rather fissured hypotympanum. This was usually only successful in non-inflamed middle ears. According to reports in the literature it should have been technically possible to measure the mucociliary beat frequency by means of a phototransistor on the microscope.

However this method was deliberately rejected since the larynx was the area of interest. On the other hand, it was not technically possible to achieve a view of the ciliary bearing subglottic or tracheal areas using the operating microscope. A right-angled view of the mucosa would only have been possible during endoscopy of the larynx under anaesthesia using a small mirror. Observation of the ciliary beat frequency under the microscope would have been technically possible after external opening of the larynx, but would have been complicated by uncertainty due to drying of the preparation and the effect of local or systemic drugs, so that accurate quantitative assessment could not have been achieved.

Therefore in vivo recording of the mucociliary activity was not used for investigation of laryngeal carcinoma. Furthermore the first step in the pathogenesis of a laryngeal carcinoma is metaplasia which could only manifest by a slight change in mucociliary activity. There appeared to be no prospect of eliminating these changes from the methodological errors.

11.2. Investigations of Mucociliary Transport Using the Saccharin Test

The saccharin test was used for the assessment of nasal mucociliary transport as recommended by Andersen et al. [21]. Powdered saccharin mixed with 5% indigo blue was used as the marker. Indigo blue is a food dye permitted in the German Federal Republic. Saccharin is no longer accepted as being carcinogenic so that it can be used as a food, or as a supplement in cough medicines.

Initially the saccharin was ground down to particles 10–20 μm in size, on the basis that this would produce less mechanical load on the mucosa. This powder was not very practicable for introduction into the nose since it adhered too firmly to the instruments in the moist environment. Therefore, a powder with a particle size of 20–50 μm was later adopted. Initial concern about any mechanical alteration was modified in the light of a personal observation by Andersen who applies a saccharin crystal about 1 mm^3 to the nasal mucosa.

The saccharin powder was picked up from a container using a moistened cotton wool probe, a nasal speculum was introduced and several particles placed on the medial surface of the inferior turbinate. The point of application lay 1–1.5 cm posterior to the anterior end of the turbinate, to ensure that the investigation was carried out in an area of ciliary epithelium. The side of the nose in the patent phase of the nasal cycle was used, as determined by questioning and inspection.

For practical purposes, the end point was the appreciation of taste in the throat by the patient. The appearance of blue stain in the nasopharynx was only used in exceptional cases.

The time between the application of the saccharin and the appreciation of taste was measured. If no taste was observed after 30 min, the saccharin was then applied directly to the tongue to exclude a disorder of taste. During the test the patient was asked to keep his head upright and to breathe freely through the nose.

This test was carried out on 20 patients with normal noses. The median duration of transit was 9 min 12.5 s (SD ± 146 s).

In designing the test we were concerned that the movement of the saccharin powder might be due to convection by the airstream. It was conceivable that the inspiratory stream would be more powerful because of the particular aerodynamics of the nose. Therefore we repeated the test on the same day at intervals of several hours in the same patients. After application of the saccharin the nose was closed with a clamp under otherwise identical conditions. The mean transit time was then prolonged to 15 min 31 s (SD ± 460 s). A significant difference was confirmed by the sign test, Wilcoxon's test and the Student's t test [88].

Since the saccharin was transported although the nose was closed it is justifiable to assume that this is an effect of the mucociliary clearance mechanism. The marked retardation of transit could be explained by the concept of Lucas and Douglas [251] that evaporation from the mucosal surface is reduced in deficient ventilation. It may be suspected that a disturbance in the carefully balanced two-layered mucous system will be produced, leading to a thicker periciliary sol layer due to increased fluid. Partial decoupling of the mucociliary system can thus be explained. Restriction of the mucociliary transport by deficient ventilation is significant in the genesis of diseases of the nose and paranasal sinuses, and conforms with the clinical observation that nasal obstruction often leads to disease of the sinuses.

A further point about the method of the saccharin test is as follows: the saccharin is used in the form of saccharinate which is highly soluble in water. Application of this substance to the mucosa causes a local rise of osmolarity. Without doubt this might disturb the equilibrium of the mucous layer, and lead to failure of the method. This phenomenon has already been observed with hygroscopic powders [24], and the value of an inert marker substance has been stressed [55, 100, 326]. Substances such as charcoal powder and ion exchange resin particles are tasteless so that either an isotope marker or continuous inspection of the pharynx is necessary for assessment.

The pure saccharin base is much less soluble in water. Sadly, local necrosis of the mucosa was found after application of this substance to a freshly removed dog's larynx, so that it was not used further.

We coupled this saccharin molecule to an ion exchange resin to produce a sweet-tasting but largely inert marker. A chromatograph column with the ion exchange resin Dowex 1-chloride, 1 × 4–100 cross linkage 4% and dry mesh 50–100 was eluted with a watery sodium saccharinate solution. The resulting product was washed several times with water, alcohol and ether and finally dried in a high vacuum. Under the microscope this substance showed no aggregation, and a particle size of 80–285 µm. Some particles of this preparation tasted sweet. Obviously the steric molecular arrangement responsible for taste is not concealed or prevented by coupling to the ion exchange resin. This material was applied to a freshly removed canine larynx to test its suitability for mucociliary transit. It was transported in the previously observed manner and speed.

This marker substance was used on 20 test subjects for the saccharin test. The mean transit time was 10 min 12.5 s, and the subjects were able to identify the sweet taste of the end point well [86]. This new substance can therefore be recommended as a marker for the saccharin test. Although dissociation of the saccharin molecules from the binding to the resin appears to be possible, the balance of flow is mainly towards the bound condition. The marker thus has the valuable advantage that it is largely inert. Furthermore it requires no particular instruments such as the gamma camera. The advantages of the isotope method and the saccharin test are combined, and the disadvantages of each eliminated with this new substance.

As is well known from the literature, and as was also obvious in our own investigations, the range of variation of the saccharin test was quite high in normal subjects. Thus it proved suitable for the diagnosis of nasal mucociliary transport disorders in various diseases of the nose and paranasal sinuses. However, the reactions of the ciliary epithelium of the upper and lower respiratory tracts cannot be compared with each other in oncological investigations since the appropriate injurious agent is inhaled orally and thus bypasses the upper respiratory tract before reaching the larynx. Therefore the saccharin test did not appear suitable for investigating the larynx, and was not used further.

11.3. Cytological Investigation by Measurement of the Ciliary Beat Frequency in vitro

Quantitative measurements of the ciliary activity using cytological observation of viable ciliary epithelium have been reported frequently. Therefore it appeared worthwhile to use this apparently sensitive method for oncological problems.

The culture medium was based on a Hank's solution free of sodium bicarbonate and buffered with Hepes buffer. This entire solution was adjusted with 1 N sodium hydroxide to a pH value of 7.35, and filtered by sterile methods [228].

Viable ciliary epithelium was taken from the nose of the conscious patient without local anaesthesia; the subject occasionally experienced itching or even sneezing. No damage or bleeding was caused in more than 100 procedures.

A nylon brush mounted on a thin steel wire with a diameter of about 2 mm, similar to that used for taking cytological smears during bronchoscopy, was used for obtaining cellular material.

The cytological specimen can also be obtained with a curette. This technique was not used since it must be carried out under vision with the nasal speculum, and is thus more time consuming.

The brush was introduced for a distance of 4–6 cm into the nose parallel to the inferior turbinate, moved back and forth, rotated and then removed. Simultaneous inspection ensured that material was harvested from the nasal septum, the floor of the nose or the medial surface of the inferior turbinate. Ciliary epithelium is normally found in this area. Introduction of the brush into the inferior meatus increases the cell yield but is not tolerated without local anaesthesia. Also, the cell yield is increased if the brush is first smeared with saline solution. A specimen can be taken with the brush during endoscopy of the trachea after a tracheotomy or laryngectomy.

Directly after taking the specimen, the brush is agitated about 20 times in 100 µl of the culture solution which is warmed in a water bath at 37 °C. The well of a specially ground slide is immediately filled with this cell solution and then covered with a coverslip to protect against drying. The slide was first warmed to 37 °C. The resulting culture chamber with a plano-convex volume has a maximum depth of about 720 µm, occasionally producing thick cell layers which are difficult to assess by microscopy.

For this reason the cell suspension after mixing was put in a prewarmed conventional Fuchs-Rosenthal counting chamber. The movement of the ciliary cells was not inhibited at a chamber depth of 200 µm. On the other hand, the depth of the chamber made quantitative assessment easy. The disadvantage of this preparation technique was drying, which makes assessment of the preparation within 20 min mandatory. The preparation was examined under a phase contrast microscope mounted on a Zeiss Universal microscope at magnifications between 100 and 1,000 diameters (see fig. 10).

The microscopic stage was maintained at a temperature of 37 °C, using a thermostatically controlled heating which had been constructed personally. In this way viable ciliary epithelial cells could be observed alone, or in clumps, showing easily visible ciliary activity. In addition cil-

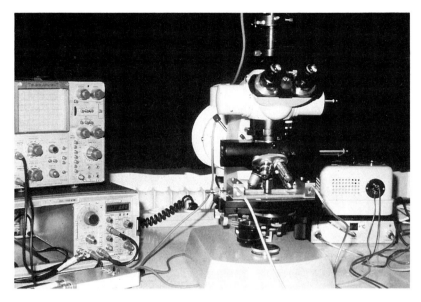

Fig. 10. Photometry apparatus and microscope with objective table capable of being heated.

iary epithelium with cytoplasmic protrusions were found which were regarded as signs of cell death [281]. Squamous cells, too, were found.

In order to determine the ciliary frequency of viable cells in this preparation a photometric apparatus was attached to the microscope as follows (see fig. 11).

The observation beam was divided by a beam splitter, and then led into a newly constructed tube. An aperture changer was introduced into the focal plane so that diaphragms with a diameter down to 250 μm could be introduced. A photo-transistor (BPX 25) was mounted behind the diaphragm.

The variations in voltage produced by illumination of the photo-transistor were amplified without filtration by a self-constructed pre-amplifier and the amplifying part of a band pass filter AF, 501 (Tektronix). The resulting signal was conducted through the low-pass Rockland System 815 filter with a limiting frequency of 40 Hz. It was then further amplified in the amplification part of a band pass filter (Tektronix AF 501) and then displayed on a storage oscilloscope (Telequipment DM 64) with the appropriate sweep frequency.

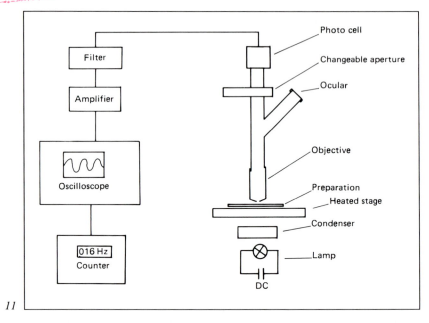

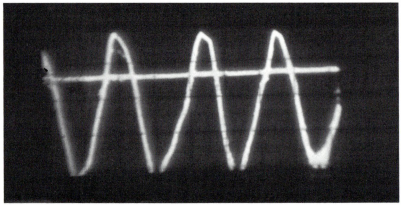

Fig. 11. Diagram of microscope – photometry apparatus.
Fig. 12. Wave on the oscilloscope with trigger threshold marked.

A digital counter (Tektronix DC 503) was bridge-connected at a fixed amplification ratio to the oscilloscope, and the counting threshold regulated to a known and marked amplitude height on the oscilloscope screen (see fig. 12).

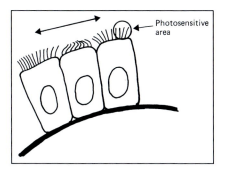

Fig. 13. Correct adjustment of the measuring field on fixed cells.

Initially the microscope was driven by a personally constructed direct-current source. However it turned out that the main frequency in the light meter attachment was largely eliminated by the low pass filter, even under amplification, so that 50 Hz alternating current could be used. For measurement of the ciliary frequency an active cell was introduced into the photometric measuring area, and marked with an eyepiece micrometer so that the rhythmic movements of the ciliary border caused changes in light intensity. These changes in light intensity were then demonstrated on the oscilloscope as a wave pattern which could be measured under appropriate amplification when the threshold was exceeded. The counting interval was 1 s, so that the frequency could be read off directly in Hz.

Only those cells were counted whose cell bodies were fixed, and which thus produced movement of the cilia alone. Individual active cells lying free in the solution were difficult to hold for long enough in the photometric measuring area. Furthermore it must be taken into account that in the presence of oscillating cell bodies the resulting total frequency of the cilia-cell complex is co-determined by the mass of the cell body by resonance effects (see fig. 13).

Moreover the waves on the oscilloscope were clearer, more sinusoidal and freer from distortion, the smaller the measuring surface. A spot size of 2 µm was thus chosen with appropriate magnification and choice of diaphragm. Tracings recorded from larger measuring surfaces included superimposition due to the activity of several cells.

The assessment of the tracings on the oscilloscope generates further problems in that intermediate waves must be assessed in the presence of irregular tracings. The amplification should be chosen so that only tracings which are regarded as representing ciliary activity exceed the counting threshold.

In order to get an overview of the effectiveness of the removal of the specimen from the nose a preparation was made as already described in a counting chamber. The cells were counted using a hand-counting apparatus (Instrumentation Laboratory, Leucodiff 700) and classified as viable or non-viable ciliated epithelial cells and squamous cells.

A pilot series on 19 subjects showed that the assessment of vital cytological smears should be carried out as quickly as possible. Since antibiotics were not added to the culture solution to avoid their pharmacological effects a visible bacterial colonisation developed within about 1 h. The ciliary frequency was less during later measurements, and the proportion of viable ciliary epithelial cells decreased markedly after 2–4 h.

An experiment was also carried out in which nasal cytological smears were taken on successive days from 19 subjects. Since there was neither subjective nor objective change in the patients' symptoms within this short period of time this series serves for assessment of reproducibility. There were occasional differences in the total cell count and in the proportion of viable ciliary cells, so that it appears advisable not to over-estimate the significance of a single finding [84].

The sensitivity of the method was tested by taking smears from the trachea of 18 patients who had undergone a tracheotomy or a laryngectomy more than 4 weeks previously. This experiment showed a much higher proportion of squamous cells, supporting the concept of metaplasia of the tracheal epithelium due to direct exposure to air [87].

Since varying ciliary frequencies can almost always be recorded from different cells in cytological specimens there are methodological problems with assessment of this finding. Therefore, we attempted to make ten measurements at different points on the most active cell specimen to arrive at a mean value. Also measurement at one point during 30 s showed variations of the ciliary frequency measured over a period of 1 s of up to ± 2 Hz so that evaluation is needed for each individual cell.

Stroboscopy was also tried for measurement of ciliary frequency and observation of the ciliary beat. The cytological specimen as described above was placed on a heated table of a Zeiss Universal microscope. Illumination was provided by a Xenon flash conducted by a mirror into the illumination beam of the microscope. The Xenon lamp with the appropriate flash generator is normally intended for laryngostroboscopy. For the present purpose an inbuilt trigger input on the flash generator was controlled by the model 405 Systron Donner function generator. Flash frequencies down to 5 Hz could thus be produced by adjusting the generator.

Observation of the specimen under illumination by the stroboscope was easily possible. However immediately the flash frequency was lower than 18 Hz (that is the eye's fusion frequency) a continuous image was no longer observed. This made observation difficult and very tiring. Even when using multiples of the supposed ciliary frequency a slow-motion or virtual standstill could not be observed. In addition to the variations of frequency within seconds, and a non-uniform frequency in the specimen as a whole, stroboscopy failed because an individual cilium is seldom observed in a cytological smear. During observation of a ciliary border there is always a phase difference determined by the metachronous nature of the beat. Since the ciliary speed differs within the various beat phases, stroboscopic observation at such low frequencies is difficult. For this reason the method was abandoned for cytological assessment.

Cytological smears were taken from the subglottic area of 10 patients undergoing laryngectomy. The individual patients are illustrated later, in the series of laryngectomies. In larynges in which mucociliary transport could be recorded, active ciliary cells were also found in the cytological smear. The ciliary frequency was measured on as many cells as possible, up to a maximum of 10. It showed an intra-individual variation averaging 4 Hz. In the inter-individual comparison ciliary frequency was spread over a large physiological range of 6–18 Hz. Due to this considerable variation a statistical analysis with mean values did not appear to be valid for this purpose.

Cytological smears were also taken from larynges which showed no mucociliary transport. In cases in which no ciliary activity was visible using the reflex method under the operating microscope, no active ciliary cells were to be found in cytological smears either. Active cells were also found in the smear from an irradiated larynx without mucociliary transit but with visible ciliary activity.

A picture of the condition of the mucosa can be obtained by cell differentiation of the cytological smear. Development of this aspect may be more promising for further studies than single frequency measurements.

Because of the methodological problems already addressed, the cytological smear was not used further for the investigation of larynges removed for cancer. The method of cytological smears appeared not to be sensitive enough for investigation of oncological problems in the larynx. Displacement of cell differentiation in the smear appeared to be of more

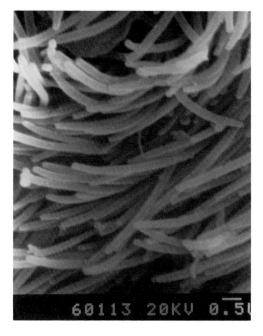

Fig. 14. Ciliary blanket under the scanning electron microscope (× 12,800).

interest in carcinogenesis than change in ciliary frequency. However, procuring material from the larynx, and especially from the subglottic space without anaesthesia appeared to be more difficult.

11.4. Electron Microscopy

Directly after removal, a fresh specimen was fixed in 2% glutaraldehyde, buffered to pH 7.3 with Sorensen-phosphate buffer. The buffer solution was then washed out, the specimen fixed in 1% osmium tetroxide and dehydrated in a series of alcohols of increasing concentration. For scanning electron microscopy the specimen was sputtered with a gold layer, after critical point drying. Scanning electron microscopy was carried out on the Hitachi S 450 apparatus.

Further processing for transmission microscopy was carried out by embedding in epoxy resin after further dehydration in propylene glycol.

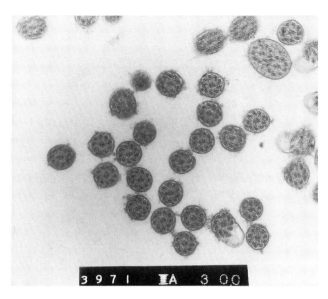

Fig. 15. Ciliary section under the transmission electron microscope (× 28,500). The direction of the central tubules should be noted. Giant cilia can be seen to the right and above.

Ultra-thin sections were placed on a copper mesh and counter-stained with lead citrate and uranyl acetate. The investigation was carried out on the Zeiss EM 9S2 or the Hitachi H 500 electron microscope.

A pilot study was carried out first on operative material taken from the nasal mucosa. The cilia were easy to demonstrate both by scanning and transmission electron microscopy (fig. 14, 15), whereas the ultrastructural details of the axonemata, the dynein arms and radial spokes could not be demonstrated with certainty (fig. 16). However the figures reproduced in the literature were not appreciably clearer, so that great efforts were not made in this respect.

During the operation, specimens were taken for scanning and transmission electron microscopy from the lateral tracheal wall about 3 cm inferior to the free edge of the vocal cord from 6 patients undergoing laryngectomy for carcinoma.

The findings were as follows: The epithelium was not regularly visible in scanning electron microscopy, since large parts of the surface were cov-

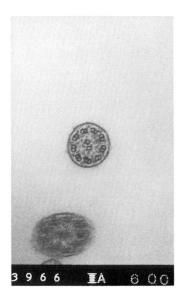

3 9 6 6   ⅡA   6 00

Fig. 16. Transverse section of a cilium with partially visible dynein arms (× 57,000).

ered by a firmly adherent layer of mucus, fibrin and erythrocytes (fig. 17). The epithelium varies from patient to patient, in some showing epithelium of normal thickness and cilia arranged in one direction (fig. 18), and in some a surface formed by squamous epithelium (fig. 19) or quite often a layer of basal cells which carried many microvilli on their surface (fig. 20).

Ciliary epithelial cells and basal cells with microvilli were often found in proximity (fig. 20).

Occasionally an increased extrusion of ciliary cells from the epithelial units was visible, as well as a decrease of cells and loosening of cell connections in the area of squamous epithelium (fig. 21, 22). These phenomena have also been reported in the literature [211, 237, 253, 406, 407, 436]. A crest formation was found on the surface of fixed squamous epithelial units, as is already known from findings in the squamous epithelium of the vocal cord [237].

Fig. 17. Mucus, fibrin and erythrocytes lying on the epithelium (× 1,100).
Fig. 18. Correctly lying ciliary epithelium (× 2,550).
Fig. 19. Squamous epithelial surface (× 10,200).
Fig. 20. Basal cell with microvilli (× 2,550).

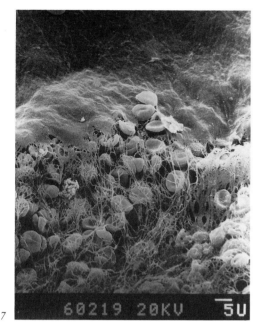

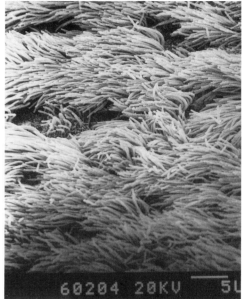

17

18

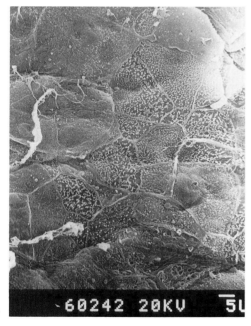

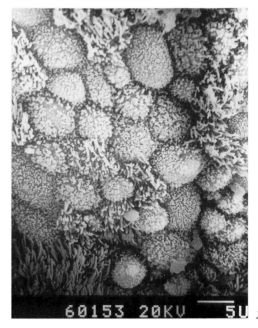

19

20

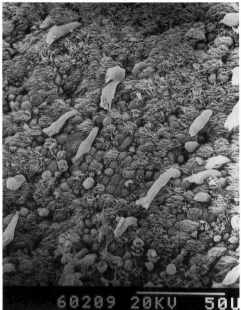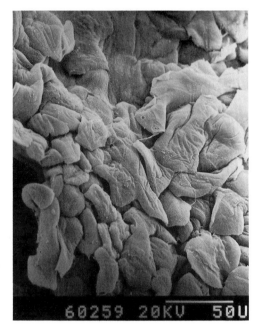

Fig. 21. Extrusion of ciliary cells (× 600).
Fig. 22. Withdrawal of squamous epithelial cells (× 510).

It was also difficult to demonstrate dynein arms by transmission microscopy with certainty. In one specimen, cilia were found with clearly visible arms, in addition to axenomata which were clearly without dynein.

In patients in whom scanning electron microscopy had shown basal cells carrying microvilli, transmission microscopy showed many microvilli in addition to cilia (fig. 23).

Increased aberration in the arrangement of the direction of the central tubules was not found (fig. 15). Numerical aberrations of the tubules and giant cilia were often demonstrated (fig. 15, 24).

In summary, electron microscopy of the subglottic area in patients with laryngeal carcinoma showed metaplasia of the ciliary epithelium of variable extent. The ciliary epithelium was replaced by a basal cell layer of squamous epithelium. Also the ultrastructure of the axonemata of the cilia demonstrated numerical aberrations of the tubules and giant cilia which can be attributed to a continuous inflammatory stimulus or to an external noxious agent.

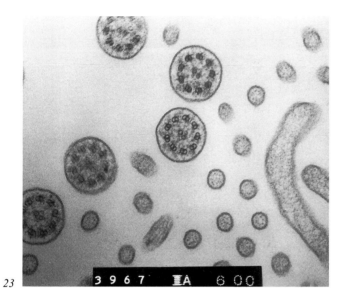

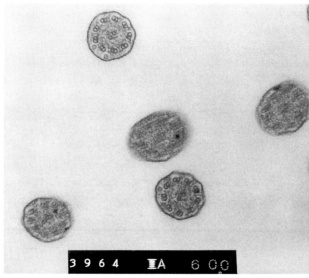

Fig. 23. Section of cilia and microvilli (× 57,000).
Fig. 24. Numerical aberrations of microtubules (× 57,000).

12. Investigations of Mucociliary Transport in Human Larynges Removed for Carcinoma

12.1. Method

Physiological investigations of the ciliary epithelium of larynges affected with cancer were attempted. Initially, freshly removed larynges were examined immediately under the operating microscope at magnifications up to 20 diameters. In the subglottic space, ciliary activity was often visible from the light reflex. The viability of the epithelium persisted after the cessation of circulation, after the larynx has been removed and also after alterations due to operative manipulations and intubation anaesthesia. Therefore a culture chamber was constructed which enabled continuous observations to be made at 37 °C and with high humidity. This type of investigation has not so far been described in the literature. For this investigation we used a Plexiglas water bath with a thermostatically controlled suspended heating apparatus made by Julabo (fig. 25).

A chrome-nickel (Nirosta) tank was suspended in the bath so that it was immersed in the water which was heated to 37 °C. The specimen tank was closed off from the external air, and covered with a glass pane so that a saturated atmosphere could be produced over the specimen. A Zeiss OpMi I operating microscope was used for the observations. A 35 mm Canon camera was attached to the microscope with a beam splitter. Photographs were taken using 160 ASA artificial light film, at an aperture of 64 and an exposure time between 1 and 5 s.

Larynges freshly removed in the operating room were placed in a thermal transport vessel, at 37 °C with a saturated atmosphere, immediately after removal and inspection by the surgeon. They were then transported as quickly as possible in the culture chamber. The ciliary activity was observed in the laboratory with the operating microscope.

A marking substance must be used to demonstrate the mucociliary transport. Pilot studies were carried out on dogs' larynges as already described for the saccharin test. Indian ink appeared to be the most suitable of all the substances tested, such as aluminum dust, charcoal powder, methylene blue solution and ion exchange resin particles. Application of

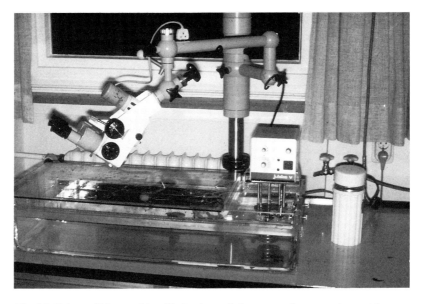

Fig. 25. Culture dish, capable of being heated, for mucosal preparations with operating microscope and transport vessel on the right hand side.

the ink did not breach the mucous layer, and the pathway due to transit of the ink could be well seen and photographed by following the streaks made by the ink.

After preliminary experiments with pipettes and capillary tubing, it appeared that dots of ink of appropriate size were produced most practically with a marking pen made by Rotring whose point had a diameter of 0.13 mm.

One or more rings of dots were made 0.5–3 cm apart in the subglottic space of freshly removed larynges (fig. 26, 27).

The onset of transit of the dots was observed and photographed. The transit speed usually lay between 1 and 5 mm/min, so that the entire observation time of the subglottic space was about 15 min.

In individual cases transit was considerably slower, in which case observation was prolonged to a maximum of 2 h, with photographic recording. Transit was not visible in all larynges, as is clear in the results. Sometimes a larynx had first to be freed from a thick layer of blood and mucus, using a cotton wool probe, before mucociliary transport could be demonstrated.

In specimens with good transport the larynx was carefully wiped after the transit was completed, and new dots were created. In some cases mucociliary transit then resumed. If a larynx showed no mucociliary transit after removal of tenacious mucus an attempt was made to change the consistency of the mucus by irrigation with acetylcystine solution (Mucolyticum Lappe® solution) or by spraying with a solution containing acetylcystine (Rinofluimucil S®). However, mucociliary transit could not be stimulated by these procedures in any case.

There were occasional difficulties in preparing freshly removed specimens and occasionally delays due to the necessary clinical organisation. Other larynges which had been stored for up to 3 h at room temperature in moist towels regularly demonstrated uncompromised transit function in some areas.

Since a proportion of the larynges showed no mucociliary transport despite all care during preparation, an attempt was made to carry out transit investigations during the operation. The laryngectomy was begun in one patient with immediate demonstration and opening of the trachea, reintubation of the tracheal stump and freeing of the tracheal stump on the laryngeal side. A ring of dots was then made in the subglottic space, as had previously been done in the specimens. The mucociliary transport which had occurred in the intervening period was observed after carrying out the laryngectomy in the usual manner. However, despite careful dissection, the subglottis was filled with mucus and blood after the laryngectomy so that mucociliary transport could not be observed. Thus this procedure did not appear promising.

In order to investigate whether larynges which showed neither transit nor ciliary activity demonstrated any ciliary epithelium the specimen was examined later by histology.

12.2. Results

The results of the transit investigation on 75 larynges affected with cancer will now be illustrated; these laryngectomies were carried out between June 1984 and March 1986 in the ENT Clinic of the University of Münster. The results will be illustrated using a diagram of a larynx split posteriorly and opened up (fig. 28). A larynx prepared in this way is illustrated in figure 29.

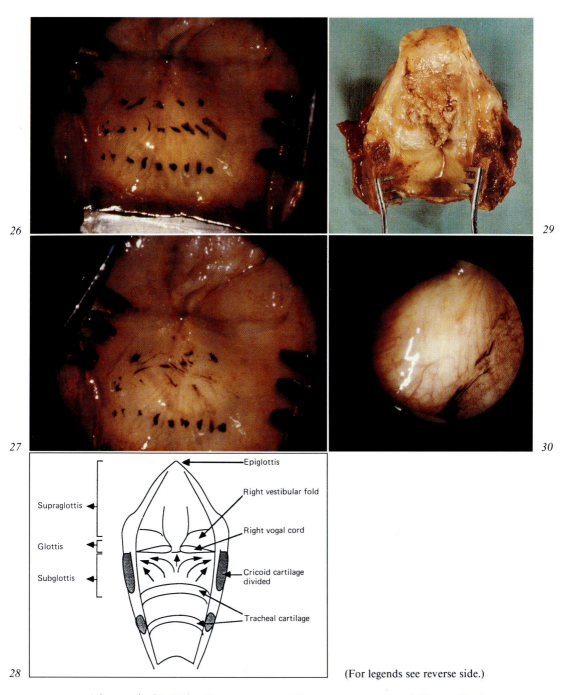

(For legends see reverse side.)

Fig. 26. Application of Indian ink to the subglottic space of an excised human larynx. Mucociliary transport is beginning on the right side.

Fig. 27. Mucociliary transport in the subglottic space (compare with fig. 26).

Fig. 28. Diagram of the larynx with marked mucociliary transport ways.

Fig. 29. Human larynx opened posteriorly.

Fig. 30. Endoscopic view into the left subglottic space with mucociliary transport pathway rendered visible by streaks of Indian ink on the lower edge of the vocal cord. Part of the tracheal tube can be seen below.

The anatomical details and regions are given in the following diagrams. Furthermore the directions of the normal mucociliary transit are indicated by arrows. Mucociliary transport cannot be demonstrated in the supraglottic area either of man or animals, as far as we know.

An arrow is used to indicate mucociliary transport in those larynges where it was present. The tumour area is shown hatched, and the pT and pN stage and the histology of the tumour are also indicated. A distant metastasis was not demonstrated in any patient.

Unless specifically stated, patients had not undergone tracheotomy or irradiation before the laryngectomy. If the mucociliary transport was reproducible or ciliary activity was present in a patient without mucociliary transport this is also stated. In those cases in which the ciliary beat frequency was determined this is also recorded.

For the patients in whose larynx mucociliary transport was no longer visible after the larynx had been removed the data are summarised in table 2 on page 89 to save space.

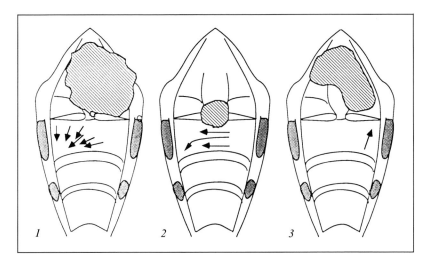

Patient 1: A.F., 74-year-old man. Well differentiated keratinising squamous cell carcinoma, pT4 pNO, mucociliary transport reproducible.

Patient 2: B.H., 70-year-old man. Well differentiated keratinising squamous cell carcinoma, pT3 pNO, mucociliary transport reproducible.

Patient 3: B.K., 53-year-old man. Poorly differentiated non-keratinising squamous cell carcinoma, pT3 pN1.

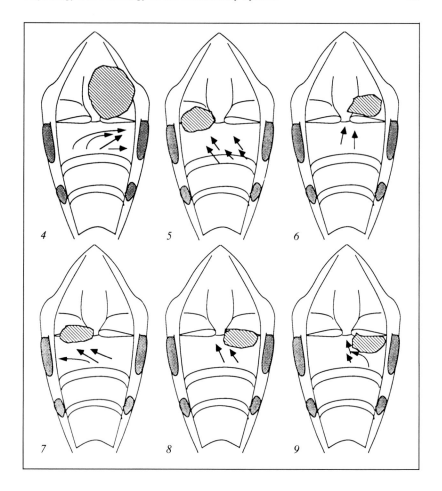

Patient 4: B.W., 56-year-old man. Slightly keratinising squamous cell carcinoma, pT3 pN1, mucociliary transport reproducible, ciliary beat frequency 13–17 Hz.

Patient 5: D.B., 40-year-old man. Keratinising squamous cell carcinoma, pT3 pNO, ciliary beat frequency 8–12 Hz.

Patient 6: D.A., 56-year-old woman. Papillary, squamous cell carcinoma, pT3 pNO.

Patient 7: D.W., 53-year-old man. Well differentiated keratinising squamous cell carcinoma, pT3 pNO.

Patient 8: E.R., 73-year-old woman. Keratinising squamous cell carcinoma, pT3 pNO.

Patient 9: F.E., 67-year-old woman. Keratinising squamous cell carcinoma, pT2 pNO.

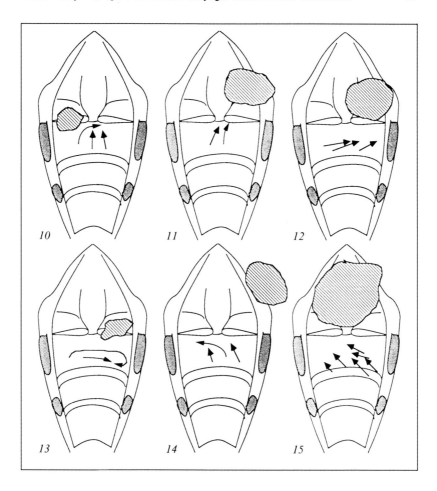

Patient 10: F.A., 82-year-old man. Previously irradiated, keratinising squamous cell carcinoma, corresponding to pT3 pNO.

Patient 11: G.J., 43-year-old man. Papillomatous, partly well and partly poorly differentiated squamous cell carcinoma, pT4 pN1, mucociliary transport reproducible.

Patient 12: G.F., 56-year-old man. Poorly differentiated slightly keratinising squamous cell carcinoma, pT3 pNO.

Patient 13: H.W., 72-year-old man. Keratinising squamous cell carcinoma. pT2 pNO.

Patient 14: H.E., 46-year-old man. Moderately differentiated keratinising squamous cell carcinoma, pT2 pNO, mucociliary transport reproducible, ciliary beat frequency 8–12 Hz.

Patient 15: H.H., 63-year-old man. Keratinising squamous cell carcinoma, pT4 pNO, mucociliary transport reproducible.

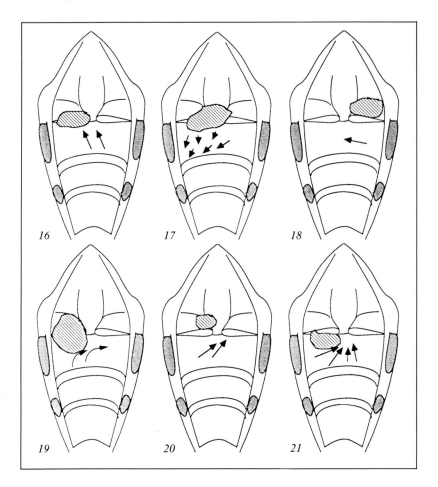

Patient 16: H.I., 54-year-old woman. Papillomatous poorly differentiated non-keratinising squamous cell carcinoma, pT2 pNO.

Patient 17: H.J., 63-year-old man. Non-keratinising squamous cell carcinoma, pT2 pNO, mucociliary transport reproducible.

Patient 18: I.C., 42-year-old woman. Poorly differentiated keratinising squamous cell carcinoma, pT3 pNO.

Patient 19: K.K.R., 45-year-old man. Well differentiated keratinising squamous cell carcinoma, pT4 pNO, mucociliary transport reproducible.

Patient 20: K.H., 54-year-old man. Moderately differentiated squamous cell carcinoma, pT1b pN1.

Patient 21: K.J., 69-year-old man. Poorly differentiated keratinising squamous cell carcinoma, pT3 pNO.

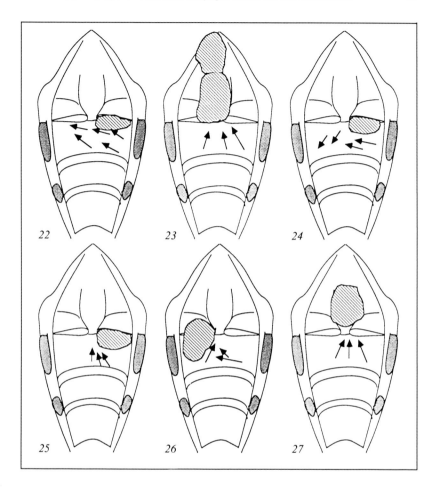

Patient 22: K.K., 51-year-old man. Well differentiated keratinising squamous cell carcinoma, pT2 pNO, mucociliary transport reproducible.

Patient 23: L.K., 71-year-old woman. Well differentiated papillary squamous carcinoma, pT4 pNO.

Patient 24: L.A., 52-year-old man. Slightly keratinised squamous cell carcinoma, pT3 pNO, mucociliary transport reproducible.

Patient 25: L.A., 51-year-old man. Keratinised squamous cell carcinoma. pT3 pNO, mucociliary transport reproducible.

Patient 26: M.H., 71-year-old man. Previous tracheotomy, keratinising squamous cell carcinoma, pT3 pNO, mucociliary transport reproducible, ciliary beat frequency 9–14 Hz.

Patient 27: M.K., 58-year-old man. Keratinising squamous cell carcinoma, pT1 pNO, mucociliary transport reproducible.

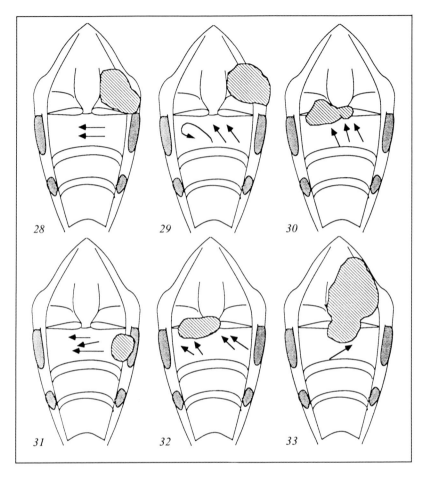

Patient 28: M.K., 61-year-old man. Small cell carcinoma, pT2 pNO, mucociliary transport reproducible, ciliary beat frequency 11–13 Hz.

Patient 29: N.E., 61-year-old man. Poorly differentiated non-keratinising squamous cell carcinoma, pT4 pNO, mucociliary transport reproducible, ciliary beat frequency 6–18 Hz.

Patient 30: P.W., 55-year-old man. Well differentiated keratinising squamous cell carcinoma, pT2 pNO, mucociliary transport reproducible.

Patient 31: P.H., 66-year-old man. Surgery and irradiation for a bronchial carcinoma 4 years previously, small cell poorly differentiated squamous cell carcinoma, pT2 pNO, mucociliary transport reproducible.

Patient 32: R.H., 79-year-old man. Previous tracheotomy, poorly keratinising squamous cell carcinoma, pT4 pNO, mucociliary transport reproducible.

Patient 33: D.B., 55-year-old man. Keratinising squamous cell carcinoma, pT3 pN1.

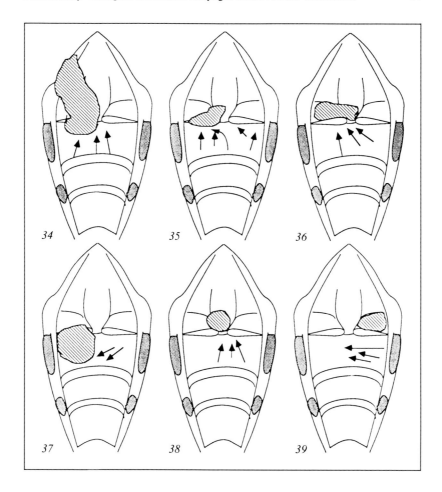

Patient 34: S.K.O., 67-year-old man. Well differentiated keratinising squamous cell carcinoma, pT4 pNO, mucociliary transport reproducible.

Patient 35: S.M., 39-year-old woman. Keratinising squamous cell carcinoma, pT2 pNO, mucociliary transport reproducible.

Patient 36: S.J., 58-year-old man. Poorly differentiated non-keratinising squamous cell carcinoma, pT1b pNO, mucociliary transport reproducible.

Patient 37: S.P., 71-year-old man. Well differentiated keratinising squamous cell carcinoma, pT2 pNO.

Patient 38: T.W., 59-year-old man. Keratinising squamous cell carcinoma, pT2 pNO, mucociliary transport reproducible, ciliary beat frequency 12–16 Hz.

Patient 39: V.W., 61-year-old man. Poorly keratinised squamous cell carcinoma, pT3 pNO.

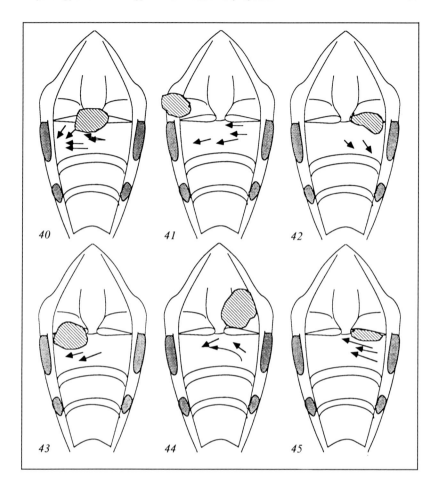

Patient 40: V.H., 65-year-old man. Keratinising squamous cell carcinoma, pT4 pNO, mucociliary transport reproducible.

Patient 41: W.F., 64-year-old man. Moderately differentiated squamous cell carcinoma, pT2 pNO, mucociliary transport reproducible.

Patient 42: W.J., 55-year-old man. Moderately differentiated squamous cell carcinoma, pT2 pNO.

Patient 43: W.W., 66-year-old man. Moderately differentiated keratinising squamous cell carcinoma, pT3 pNO, mucociliary transport reproducible.

Patient 44: Z.G., 63-year-old man. Well differentiated keratinising squamous cell carcinoma, pT1b pNO.

Patient 45: Z.G., 45-year-old man. Well differentiated keratinising squamous cell carcinoma, pT2 pNO.

Table 2. Data of patients without demonstrable laryngeal mucociliary transport

Specimen		Sex	Histology	pTN-stage	Site	Previous treatment	Ciliary activity	Li Mi
number	age, years							
46	55	M	KC	T3-NO	glott	–	yes	–
47	58	M	an Ca	T4-NO	supg	–	yes	–
48	81	M	NKC	T2-NO	glott	Rad	no	yes
49	64	M	HKC	T1-NO	supg	RadTT	no	yes
50	74	M	PDC	T2-NO	supg	–	no	yes
51	64	M	KC	T3-NO	supg	–	yes	–
52	57	M	KC	T3-NO	supg	–	no	no
53	44	M	KC	T1-NO	subg	TT	yes	–
54	51	M	KC	T2-NO	glott	TT	no	no
55	57	M	KC	T1-NO	glott	Rad	no	no
56	40	M	KC	T3-NO	supg	Rad	no	no
57	58	M	HKC	T1-NO	subg	–	no	no
58	63	M	HKC	T3-NO	supg	–	no	no
59	40	M	KC	T4-N3	supg	–	yes	–
60	60	M	KC	T2-NO	supg	–	no	yes
61	80	M	HKC	T4-NO	glott	Rad	no	yes
62	74	M	KC	T4-NO	glott	Rad	yes	–
63	44	M	an Ca	T2-NO	supg	–	no	yes
64	64	M	KC	T2-NO	supg	–	no	no
65	65	M	KC	T3-NO	glott	–	yes	–
66	61	M	KC	T4-NO	glott	Rad	no	no
67	64	M	KC	T3-N1	glott	–	no	yes
68	40	M	HKC	T3-NO	supg	–	no	no
69	50	M	HKC	T2-NO	glott	Rad	yes	–
70	80	M	KC	T3-NO	glott	–	no	no
71	62	M	NKC	T2-NO	glott	–	yes	–
72	72	F	KC	T2-NO	glott	–	yes	–
73	51	M	KC	T1-NO	glott	Rad	yes	–
74	64	M	KC	T4-NO	supg	–	no	no
75	63	M	NKC	T3-NO	supg	–	no	no

Histology: KC = keratinising squamous cell carcinoma; NKC = non-keratinising squamous cell carcinoma; HKC = highly differentiated, keratinising, squamous cell carcinoma; PDC = poorly differentiated squamous cell carcinoma; an Ca = anaplastic carcinoma.
pTN stage by the UICC classification.
Site: glott = glottic, supg = supraglottic, subg = subglottic.
Previous treatment: Rad = radiotherapy, TT = tracheotomy.
Ciliary activity: Was ciliary activity visible under the operating microscope?
Li Mi: Was ciliary epithelium visible under light microscopy?

13. Investigations of the Normal Laryngeal Mucociliary Transport

Further investigations were carried out to obtain personal data about the normal course of mucociliary transport to supplement the evidence available in the literature.

13.1. Postmortem Material

Investigations were carried out to demonstrate mucociliary transport on the dead. This investigation appeared promising, since Messerklinger [283] had obtained data about mucociliary transport in the paranasal sinuses using cadavers. However, no mucociliary transport could be demonstrated in laryngeal specimens taken at postmortem. Mucociliary transport could no longer be demonstrated in a patient who was subjected to postmortem three days after death, although a cytological smear showed the presence of some viable ciliary cells. Thus, it was suspected that the failure of transit investigations was mainly due to postmortem changes in the mucous layer. The deterioration of the disease process, often requiring endotracheal intubation, and the frequent pneumonia and bronchitis of moribund patients offer an obvious explanation.

Laryngeal observations on organ explants of clinically dead patients was rapidly rejected because of legal difficulties, and also because of prior long-term endotracheal intubation.

13.2. Subglottoscopy

Transconioscopy has produced data about ciliary transit in the subglottic area. However, we use Kleinsasser's method of microlaryngoscopy in our clinic rather than this method. We believe that transconioscopy in addition to transoral endoscopy is only indicated in special circumstances, for example a suspected subglottic carcinoma, because of the further burden for the patient. It was thus not possible to gather even approximately normal findings.

However, in our clinic microlaryngoscopy is occasionally done for minor non-malignant lesions, for example in an attempt to improve the voice. We developed a method of investigation of ciliary transit during such a procedure. A 90° Hopkin's telescope was introduced into the larynx after endotracheal intubation and introduction of the microlaryngoscope in the usual way. The mucociliary activity could be seen from the reflected light under the magnification produced by the lens. Small ink dots were made on the mucosa of the subglottis with a blunt hook. The mucociliary transport was then observed with the telescope in the succeeding minutes. The Indian ink was completely washed away and sucked off after the experiment.

The following results were obtained:

- A 48-year-old woman (Ch.W.) underwent microlaryngoscopy for Reinke's oedema of the vocal cords. Neither ciliary activity demonstrated by the light reflex nor transit of Indian ink were demonstrated in the subglottic space.
- An 18-year-old girl (M.P.) underwent microlaryngoscopy for a small mucous retention cyst of the vestibular folds. The direction of the mucociliary transport observed is illustrated (patient 76).
- A 54-year-old woman (A.H.) underwent microlaryngoscopy for a vocal cord cyst on the right side; the glottic chink was narrow. Neither ciliary activity nor transit of Indian ink could be demonstrated in the subglottic space. The patient was found at the time of the operation to have a symptomless maxillary opacity which was interpreted as a maxillary sinusitis.
- A 36-year-old man (F.K.) underwent microlaryngoscopy for a leukoplakic polyp at the anterior end of the left vocal cord with minimal epithelial dysplasia. The direction of the mucociliary transport is illustrated (patient 77).
- A lady aged 61 (G.Sch.) underwent microlaryngoscopy for a right vocal cord polyp. There was definite ciliary activity in the subglottic space but no demonstrable mucociliary transport.
- A 5-year-old boy (M.St.) underwent microlaryngoscopy for screamers' nodes. Endoscopy of the subglottic space alongside the tube was not possible because of the danger of injury to the vocal cord.
- A 51-year-old man (F.B.) underwent microlaryngoscopy for a left vocal cord polyp. The direction of the mucociliary transport is illustrated (patient 78). The mucociliary transport was recorded endoscopically on photographs (fig. 30, plate I).
- A 45-year-old man (H.M.) underwent microlaryngoscopy for a leukoplakic polyp on the anterior part of the right vocal cord. The direction of the mucociliary transport is illustrated (patient 79).

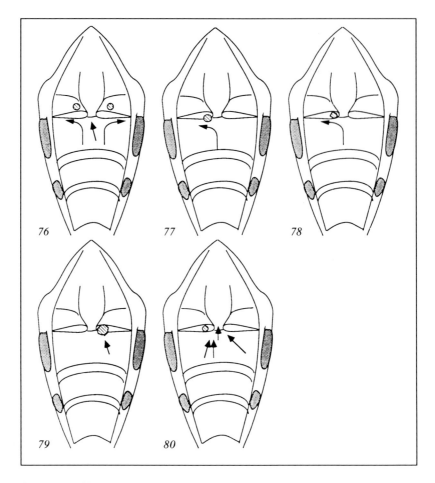

Patients 76–80. See paragraph 13.2.

In three cases the subglottis was examined during microlaryngoscopy for laryngeal carcinoma:

– A 44-year-old man (M.M.) developed an anaplastic supraglottic carcinoma on the right side. There was no evidence of ciliary activity or mucociliary transport in the subglottic space.

– A 59-year-old man (T.W.) suffered from a keratinising supraglottic squamous carcinoma on the left side. The direction of the mucociliary transport and the site of the tumour are illustrated in the following diagram. Subglottoscopy demonstrated the mucociliary transport to be in the same direction as that later found in the specimen after laryngectomy (patient 38).

- A 39-year-old man (F.-J.P.) underwent microlaryngoscopy for a keratinising squamous cell carcinoma of the anterior end of the left vocal cord. The direction of the mucociliary transit and the site of the tumour are shown (patient 80). The tumour was later removed by a frontolateral hemilaryngectomy.

13.3. The Animal Larynx

Animal experiments were carried out to obtain further data about normal laryngeal mucociliary transport.

10 cows' larynges were obtained during the normal slaughter process, about 10 min after the animal's death. They were examined about 30 min later. The mucociliary transport was demonstrated by application of Indian ink; it was present on 6 larynges. In the remaining 4 larynges only isolated ciliary activity was visible but with no transit of the Indian ink. 5 of the larynges which demonstrated transport were split posteriorly, and 1 anteriorly, and they were opened out in a special vertical stand. Axial transit was visible in the tracheal stump in the larynges opened posteriorly. When the stream reached the subglottic ledge it curved laterally and posteriorly to the right and left, continued beneath the vocal cords and then reached the posterior commissure. Spiral transit or crossing of the anterior midline were not observed (fig. 31).

In the larynx opened anteriorly, transit could be seen along the tracheal axis on the pars membranacea as far as the posterior commissure after application of Indian ink to the posterior part of the superior trachea. A marker placed laterally on the tracheal wall, once it reached the subglottic ledge, turned posteriorly under the vocal cord towards the posterior commissure. At the posterior commissure the Indian ink, along with the remnants of blood lying in the larynx, reached the area between the arytenoid cartilages, but there was no evidence of transit on the pharyngeal mucosal slope of the posterior commissure.

Investigation of the pig's larynx was also considered, but this animal is normally immersed in hot water after death before being butchered, to facilitate removal of the hair. In the opinion of the veterinary surgeon, considerable quantities of water normally gain entrance during this process, and would frustrate attempts to demonstrate mucociliary transport.

The larynges of sheep dogs and Münsterländer dogs were removed immediately after the dogs were sacrificed at the end of an experiment.

They had undergone endotracheal intubation for 3–8 h, and had been kept on the respirator in the immediately proceeding investigation. Mucociliary transport could be demonstrated in 9 of the larynges. The direction of transit was identical to that found in cattle (fig. 32).

One dog's larynx was opened anteriorly to allow the posterior commissure to be investigated. A deposit of Indian ink was found on the lateral tracheal wall inferior to the anterior third of the vocal cord. From this depot, further transit proceeded along the inferior edge of the vocal cord to the posterior commissure. When the flow reached the interarytenoid space it then turned back to the trachea at the level of the centre of the cricoid plate. Once it reached this point further transit to the interarytenoid region was recorded, so that rotatory circulation could be observed on several occasions (fig. 33).

Two larynges were also investigated during experiments on pigs. Only slight transit was recorded in both cases, mainly in the same direction as that recorded in cattle and dogs. However, ciliary streams could not be demonstrated in the same manner.

Eight rat larynges were also investigated. Abdominal operations had been carried out on these animals leading in several cases to reflux oesophagitis. Postmortem examination showed clear signs of bronchitis in several animals. Despite the smallness of the specimen, examination under the operating microscope was successful, but showed neither ciliary activity nor mucociliary transport (fig. 34).

Fig. 31. Mucociliary transport marked by Indian ink in a cow's larynx opened posteriorly.

Fig. 32. Mucociliary transport marked by Indian ink in the left half of the larynx of a dog.

Fig. 33. A dog's larynx opened anteriorly. Mucociliary transport can be seen on the inferior edge of the left vocal cord. There is circular flow at the posterior commissure.

Fig. 34. Rat's larynx stretched out with thin needles. Indian ink has been applied to the subglottic space.

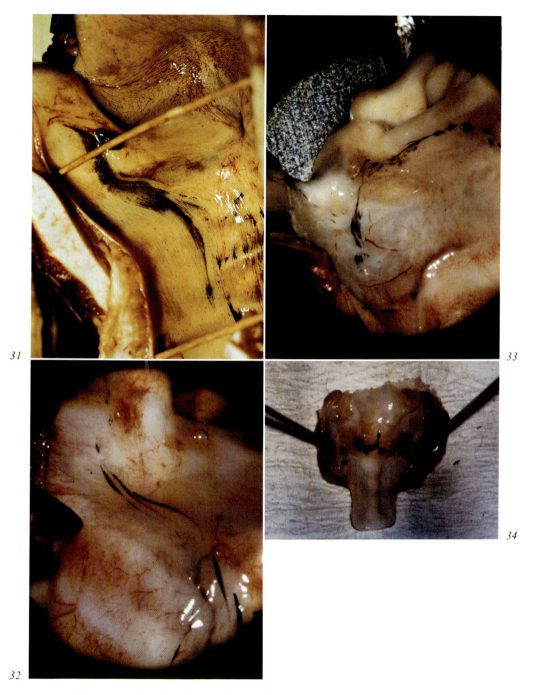

31

33

32

34

14. Discussion

14.1. Summary of the Results

Mucociliary transit was assessed in a total of 75 larynges removed for carcinoma. 39/75 (52%) were glottic and 32/75 (33%) were supraglottic tumours, the site ratio normally reported in the literature [309]. In 2 laryngeal carcinomas of the subglottic area there was no relation of the tumour to the vocal cord so that these could be classified as true subglottic carcinomas. One tumour lay in the piriform sinus, and was thus classified as a primary hypopharyngeal carcinoma.

The average age of all patients was 59.8 years at the time of laryngectomy.

The tumours were classified by the T and N system described by the UICC based on the pre-operative, intra-operative and pathological findings [441]. Clinical examination and further investigation showed no distant metastases, so that all cases were M0. Also tumours that had previously been treated by partial resection or irradiation were classified by the UICC system to record the size of the recurrent or residual tumour, but stage grouping of these previously treated tumours was not done.

Table 3 shows the results by T stage for the three specific levels of the larynx. All patients suffered from squamous carcinoma of varying degrees of differentiation. The two T_1 glottic tumours had been previously irradiated but had a residual tumour which was still T_1 in extent. In these cases therefore a laryngectomy was indicated.

Table 3. Classification related to tumour site

Site	T_1	T_2	T_3	T_4
Supraglottic	5	7	12	8
Glottic	2	15	15	7
Subglottic	2	1	–	–
Hypopharynx	–	1	–	–

Histopathological evidence of invasion of homolateral regional lymph nodes without rupture of the lymph node capsule was found in 6 of 75 (8%) of cases and was classified as pN_1. Lymphangitis carcinomatosa and extra-capsular lymph node rupture found in 1 case were classified as pN_3.

Five patients had undergone tracheotomy several days, or even months, before the laryngectomy. The laryngectomy had been preceded by radiation therapy in 10 cases.

Mucociliary transport was demonstrable in the subglottic space of 45 of the 75 larynges (60%); in 25 cases the direction and course of the muco-ciliary transport was reproducible. After carrying out a first transit experiment, Indian ink was wiped off the larynx, and transit of further dots of Indian ink was again observed. In no case the direction of transport differed from that at the first attempt.

Ciliary activity could be observed in the subglottic space using the operating microscope in 11 cases among the 30 of the 75 larynges (40%) without demonstrable mucociliary transport.

Weak ciliary activity could be observed in small areas in the supraglottic space of some larynges, usually in the angle between the vestibular fold and the epiglottis. Mucociliary transport was never demonstrated in the supraglottic area.

Two of the 5 larynges of patients submitted to preliminary tracheostomy showed neither mucociliary transport nor ciliary activity, 1 larynx showed ciliary activity but no transit, and in 2 cases a reproducible muco-ciliary transport could be demonstrated.

In 6 of the 10 irradiated larynges neither mucociliary transport nor ciliary activity could be seen, in 3 larynges there was no transit despite the presence of visible ciliary activity, and mucociliary transport was demonstrable in only 1 larynx.

14.2. Absent Mucociliary Transport in Laryngeal Preparations

The fact that 40% of the larynges showed no mucociliary transport requires an explanation. Therefore the groups of larynges with and without transit were compared. The average age of the larynges without transit was 60 years and of those with transit was 59.6 years. Thus there was no evidence of deterioration of mucociliary transport with increasing age.

There was also no relation between the histological findings, the TNM classification and the transit.

Next, the anaesthetic records of the patients were examined for the drugs used, the type and size of the tube, and the length of intubation before removal of the larynx. These data also produced no obvious differences. Intubation was carried out routinely, and the inflatable cuff lay in the upper trachea. Damage to the subglottic ciliary epithelium by the cuff was therefore not suspected [363].

Since 37% of the larynges without transit showed ciliary activity, the total proportion of larynges with ciliary activity was 75%. Persistent ciliary activity in the absence of transit can best be explained by a pathological change of the mucous component, leading either to a periciliary sol layer which is too thick, or to a thick gel layer which has undergone unfavourable change in its visco-elasticity leading to stasis of the mucociliary transport [251]. The composition of the mucus might change under anaesthesia, for example due to the use of anticholinergics or changes in the patient's fluid balance.

The sensitivity of the mucociliary system to external changes is clearly shown by the small proportion of larynges with demonstrable transit amongst the patients who had previously undergone tracheostomy or radiotherapy. The action of ionising irradiation on the ciliary epithelium is mainly to induce metaplasia and changes in the intra-epithelial glands [17, 18, 31, 33, 110, 130, 142, 169, 257, 370]. The tracheotomy divides the larynx from the respiratory stream, so that disorders of the mucous component can arise due to the loss of the evaporating effect.

Thus there is a change of the physical properties of the laryngeal mucus, particularly the visco-elasticity. Messerklinger [282, 283] showed that increased viscosity of secretion caused a considerable change of the mucociliary transport in the drainage ducts of the frontal sinuses due to the traction phenomenon. This effect was determined by the particular anatomical situation of these efferent ducts, with narrow, neighbouring mucociliary streams running in opposite directions. In the comparatively flat specimens of the larynx, such inversions of the directions of transit are not to be suspected.

Hilding [183] demonstrated the traction phenomenon of the mucous layer in the trachea. However, transport in different directions was not seen in these experiments, as was found to some extent in excised larynges. Thus the observed changes of mucociliary transport pathways are not solely the result of altered mucous visco-elasticity. This assumption is supported by the observation that the direction of mucociliary transport remains the same after wiping the mucus from the larynx. Mucociliary transport is not demonstrable in all animal experiments [182, 183, 199, 381], but there is no explanation for this absent transit in physiological studies on normal animals. Thus the absent transit in the patients described here should be ascribed to the method, and not to disease.

Light microscopy of larynges with no evidence of ciliary activity showed at most a few ciliary bearing ciliated cells. Laryngeal carcinomas are surrounded by zones of extensive squamous metaplasia that often affects the supraglottic region but only occasionally extends widely into the subglottic space [223].

14.3. The Normal Laryngeal Mucociliary Transport

In assessing the mucociliary transport found in the larynges affected with cancer it was noticeable that transit which could be regarded as normal in the light of current knowledge could not be demonstrated in a single case.

Hilding [182–184] and Zaitsu [478] investigated normal mucociliary transport in the animal larynx. Bridger and Proctor [51, 52] carried out intravital observations with isotope methods on animals and man. Unfortunately the images recorded with the camera are difficult to interpret because of the absence of anatomical landmarks.

Ewert and Martensson [118] and Bartholomé and Karduck [37] have recorded further data about mucociliary transport gained at transconioscopy on man. My own investigations during subglottoscopy under anaesthesia on patients without laryngeal carcinoma should also be referred to. My own investigations on specimens of several animal species confirmed the laryngeal transit pattern previously described by Hilding.

The morphological investigations of Pavelka et al. [329] on the larynx and trachea of animals demonstrated similar conditions to those in man. There is very little interindividual variation of mucociliary transport in rats [291].

It is thus valid to translate the conditions of normal laryngeal mucociliary transport from animal experiments to man. In particular, they agree with data obtained on man by transconioscopy and isotopes.

The problem of obtaining normal morphological findings in man apply also to electron microscopy, since the specimen must be taken as quickly as possible after death, or operation, to prevent autolytic changes. Thus routine material from postmortems and operations are correctly excluded from assessment of normal findings [12, 44, 47, 361, 462].

We were not in a position to fulfill the prequisites for normal mucociliary transit for man [278], that is the data should be obtained without physical or chemical influences from live normal subjects. However, there is no difference in the transit direction between the living or the dead [283] although the speed of the mucociliary transport is slower in the dead [286].

A parallel series of experiments on normal subjects using the required method is obviously impossible. Therefore the concepts put forward so far by all investigators relating to the normal mucociliary transit must be accepted (fig. 28).

14.4. The Significance of Abnormal Mucociliary Transport in Larynges Affected with Cancer

The relation of mucociliary transport direction and tumour site are reported here in three categories: in 22 of 45 (48.9%) cases the mucociliary transport was directed towards the tumour; in 15 of 45 (33.3%) of cases the mucociliary transport led away from the tumour; in 8 of 45 (17.8%) of cases the mucociliary transport was in an indifferent direction in relation to the tumour.

Changes of viscosity of the mucus are unlikely to cause these deviations from normal mucociliary transport. There is also no evidence that the cilia of the human respiratory tract are relatively short-lived, so that their direction of beat can change due to an artifact, as for example is well-known of highly differentiated ciliary systems of many protozoa [254]. Also all investigations have shown that the beat of the respiratory cilia is only antiplectic and does not change to symplectic or diaplectic forms [400].

In the light of clinical experience and epidemiological data [47, 223] the pathogenesis of laryngeal carcinoma is undoubtedly tied, like that of bronchial carcinoma, to exposure to an inhaled carcinogen. Cigarette smoke is pre-eminent of the exogenous carcinogens; the polycyclic aromatic hydrocarbons are regarded as the actual causative agent [223, 224]. Quite marked regional variations in the incidence of laryngeal carcinoma are often explained on closer examination by particular traditional or religious habits which determine a particularly intensive contact with, or avoidance of, well-known carcinogens. Variations between rural and urban populations can be attributed to varying degrees of air pollution, but smoking habits also vary between town and country [272].

The nose is another part of the respiratory tract which is exposed in a high degree to atmospheric pollutants. However, cigarette smoke is mainly inhaled and exhaled through the mouth, so that the nose is less exposed to this agent. The particle size also affects the site of deposition. Adenocarcinoma of the nose and nasal sinuses is a remarkable nasal tumour that is exogenously determined [3]. Mucociliary transport was found to be retarded in a cohort study of woodworkers [2]. Clear morphological changes in the epithelium have also been confirmed after exposure to wood dust in animal experiments [154].

One part of the respiratory tract is remarkably seldom the primary site of a carcinoma, that is the trachea.

Carcinogenic substances may be deposited in the respiratory tract by two mechanisms [137], the first during inspiration at sites of turbulence, the second at sites with a defective airstream. Whereas aerodynamic effects during impaction cause the particle to be thrown onto the wall of the airway, gravity causes sedimentation at points and times when the air flow is slight. If the mucociliary transport of the bronchial system is intact the carcinogen which has penetrated to the terminal bronchioles is transported out of the lungs again and into the pharynx. This mechanism can lead to local accumulation of carcinogenic material:

1. In aerodynamic terms, the larynx is an important site of constriction of the respiratory tract.

    The main airstream passes through the posterior part of the glottis [46]. However, inhaled material is mainly precipitated, at least initially, on the anterior part of the vocal cord. Thus the site of predilection of carcinoma of the larynx could be explained by impaction of carcinogens at the first important constriction during oral inhalation of noxious agents. Post-stenotic turbulence would be expected beyond a severe stenosis of the larynx leading to deposition in the subglottic space and upper trachea.

2. Two explanations are available for the deposition on the bifurcation of the major bronchi:

    A direct impaction on the aerodynamically prominent points or an accumulation due to mucociliary transport from the bronchi which must elude a blind alley at the level of the carina [183]. Since the trachea continues without bifurcations, its mucociliary transport is very effective, with no local possibilities for the development of accumulations.

3. Mucociliary clearance prevents a sedimentation in the deep periphery of the bronchi. This fact explains why bronchial carcinoma is most common in the major bronchi [183].

Finally the mucociliary transport mechanism of the lung ending in the larynx can explain the frequency of carcinomas at the latter site in comparison with the trachea.

Hilding [183] summarised these concepts and conclusions with the sentence 'the distribution of squamous cell carcinomas suggests a relation to mucociliary transport'.

Yeates et al. [475] described isotope clearance investigations of the lungs in which a spot of high activity was found in the larynx which was then transported by swallowing into the oesophagus.

Investigation of the mucociliary transport in larynges affected with cancer fills a gap which has not so far been analysed.

A highly effective transit mechanism must be provided at the larynx, the terminus of the pulmonary clearance system. This is achieved by the special laryngeal mucociliary transport mechanism which produces an accumulation of the material at the posterior commissure. At that point ciliary epithelium is only present in the folds of the posterior commissure; therefore another mechanism must be present for the last stage of transit into the pharynx. There are no certain data on this point. However, it is possible that an effective mechanism is provided by the concertina-like epithelium, the airstream and the width of the glottis varying with the respiratory cycle, in addition to the swallowing act and clearing of the throat. We attempted to observe this mechanism during a laryngofissure under local anaesthesia, but spots of Indian ink that had been applied to the posterior commissure were not passed into the pharynx. Laryngofissure probably produces a considerable change in the aerodynamic conditions.

A critical point arises in the posterior deflection of the laryngeal mucociliary transport, below the anterior third of the vocal cord. Hilding [180] observed collections of mucus at this point. Proetz [see discussion on Hilding; 180] mentioned the increased incidence of carcinoma at this point, a fact also emphasised by others [222, 295]. Also, transit towards the anterior commissure correlates with the site of predilection for the development of carcinoma. Carcinoma of the posterior commissure is very rare, although the main mass of the clearance stream runs across this area: Hilding [184] explains this by the fact that retention of carcinogens here is prevented by rapid mucus through-put. He demonstrated the necessity for prolonged contact in carcinogenesis, in contrast to laryngeal tuberculosis, for example, an infection typically affecting the posterior part of the larynx. Furthermore, the suspected aeromechanical clearing mechanism of the posterior commissure of the larynx, unlike the mucociliary mechanism, remains undamaged by inhaled toxins.

The glottis forms a boundary, free of cilia, between the supra- and subglottic spaces. This fact requires special consideration in carcinogenesis. An accumulation of carcinogens by impaction during inspiration appears rather unlikely, especially since supraglottic carcinoma is most frequent in the angle concealed between the vestibular fold and the epiglottis [223]. Penetration of substances from the subglottic space into the supraglottic area could be explained by the often described ciliary pathway at the anterior commissure. On the other hand, radiology has shown that the vocal cords at rest are tilted superiorly, so that even the area of the inferior arcuate line contacts the vestibular fold [25]. Transfer of mucus laden with carcinogens is thus possible. This would also explain the finding that nuclides instilled in vivo into the trachea can be found later in the supraglottis [51].

Our findings of abnormal mucociliary transport pathways in larynges affected with cancer can principally be explained in two ways:

1. The accumulation of carcinogenic material may be determined by constitutionally abnormal transit.

   Camner et al. [65] investigated bronchial clearance, and Andersen et al. [21] nasal clearance of monozygotic twins. They found that the mucociliary transport was a constitutional, probably genetically, determined characteristic. Thus 'slow clearing' subjects are recognised, who may have an increased risk of bronchial carcinoma [476]. The finding of a considerably retarded mucociliary clearance function of the large airways in patients with laryngeal carcinoma before surgery also supports this concept [268].

   The fact that many cigarette smokers do not develop laryngeal or bronchial carcinoma is explained by varying susceptibility. Recently this has been ascribed to a genetically determined enzyme, aryl-hydrocarbon-hydroxylase, which takes part in the metabolism of carcinogens [23, 175, 176].

   On the other hand, Matthys et al. [263] found retarded mucociliary bronchial clearance in a group of smokers with bronchial carcinoma, compared with smokers who suffered only from chronic non-malignant bronchial diseases. They coined the term 'inborn errors of mucociliary transport'.

2. In continuing exposure to carcinogens the laryngeal mucociliary trans-
    port mechanisms are disturbed, leading to accumulation of carcino-
    gens and development of a carcinoma. Investigations of carcinogene-
    sis of surfaces originally provided with ciliary epithelium describe ini-
    tial metaplasia of the ciliary epithelium with loss of the entire ciliary
    border [36, 80, 175]. The further stages of development to carcinoma
    only occur in metaplastic epithelium. However, the question remains
    whether functional changes of the ciliary epithelium occur before
    gross morphological damage can be recognised. The effect of a chronic
    inflammatory stimulus on function, in addition to morphological
    damage to the ciliary epithelium, has been illustrated recently using
    maxillary sinusitis as a model [311]. Iravani and van As [199] also
    found disturbances in co-ordination and direction of ciliary activity in
    bronchitic rats. Also ciliary anomalies were found with greater fre-
    quency during electron microscopy of ciliary epithelium undergoing
    carcinogenesis [13, 166, 433]. These ciliary anomalies are to be
    regarded as an inappropriate cilioneogenesis, in response to inhaled
    noxious agents and infections. They can be recognised by the fact that
    on the ciliary side a continuing regeneration occurs independent of the
    cell replacement. The fact that the regenerating ciliary epithelium
    adapts its direction of beat to the surrounding conditions [250] indi-
    cates a high level of intercellular co-ordination. Thus the abnormal
    laryngeal ciliary streams found in this investigation may be the first
    indication of carcinogenesis.
    Which of the two processes is the basic cause is as difficult to deter-
mine as the question of the hen and egg.
    The concept of a primary, constitutionally disordered transport is to
be preferred, because the abnormal mucociliary transport more commonly
streams towards the tumour and because of the large co-ordinated streams
which are formed.
    Further information about the pathophysiology of the mucociliary
system in relation to carcinogenesis could be obtained by investigations
which were suitable for the in vivo high resolution demonstration of mucociliary transport in the larynx. Also the development of methods for the in
vivo measurement of ciliary activity could provide decisive information.
Thus it is possible that normal data about the physiological process in man
could be obtained.

15. Summary

After a short historical introduction, the current state of knowledge of the anatomy and physiology of the mucociliary system is reviewed. Description and discussion of the clinical and experimental methods of investigation and measurement of the mucociliary transport and of the ciliary activity then follow. Light and electron microscopy are also considered. Next, the pathology, pathophysiology and pharmacology of the mucociliary system are reported. The introduction ends with the consideration of specific diseases related to the mucociliary system, such as the immotile cilia syndrome.

The main interest of this investigation is directed to changes in the ciliary epithelium in laryngeal malignancies. Therefore the literature relevant to physiology is critically evaluated.

Pilot studies of the method used for investigating the physiology of the ciliary epithelium were mainly undertaken on the more accessible nasal mucosa as a model for ciliary epithelium.

The use of the saccharin test for demonstration of nasal mucociliary transport is thoroughly assessed and the suitability of a new, improved, marking substance was tested.

The quantification of cell types for cytological assessment of nasal smears under the phase constrast microscope was appraised. The method of determination of ciliary frequency by microphotometry was evaluated critically by a series of experiments.

The author's electron microscopic findings on ciliary epithelium taken from human larynges affected with cancer are also discussed.

After these pilot studies the method of the saccharin test and the cytological smear appeared to be unsuitable for oncological investigations. Therefore, mucociliary transport in the subglottic space of 75 human larynges excised for malignancy was investigated by the development of a suitable method. This method demonstrated abnormal mucociliary transport pathways. Investigations of the normal pathway of mucociliary transport in the larynx were obtained in animal experiments and by endoscopic investigations in man.

References

1 Abraham, W.; Sielczak, M.; Delehunt, M.W.; Marchette, J.C.; Wanner, A.: Impairment of tracheal mucociliary clearance but not ciliary beat frequency by a combination of low level ozone and sulfur dioxide in sheep. Eur. J. resp. Dis. *68:* 114–120 (1986).

2 Abraham, W.M.; Kim, C.S.; Sielczak, W.M.; Eldridge, M.; Stevenson, J.S.; Chapman, G.A.; Wanner, A.: Postnatal maturation of mucociliary function in sheep: normal development and development after injury with ozone. Am. Rev. resp. Dis. *132:* suppl. 4, A 73 (1986).

3 Acheson, E.D.; Cowdell, R.H.; Hadfield, E.; Macbeth, R.G.: Nasal cancer in woodworkers in the furniture industry. Brit. med. J. *ii:* 587–596 (1968).

4 Adler, K.B.; Wooten, O.; Dulfano, M.J.: Mammalian respiratory mucociliary clearance. Archs envir. Hlth *27:* 364–369 (1973).

5 Afzelius, B.A.: Electron microscopy of the sperm tail. Results with a new fixative. J. biophys. biochem. Cytol. *5:* 269–278 (1959).

6 Afzelius, B.A.: A human syndrome caused by immotile cilia. Science *193:* 317–319 (1976).

7 Afzelius, B.A.: The immotile cilia syndrome and other ciliary diseases. Int. Rev. exp. Path. *19:* 1–4 (1979).

8 Afzelius, B.A.: Immotile cilia syndrome and ciliary abnormalities induced by infection and injury. Am. Rev. resp. Dis. *124:* 107–109 (1981).

9 Afzelius, B.A.: Ultrastructural basis for ciliary motility. Eur. J. resp. Dis. *64:* suppl. 128, pp. 280–286 (1983).

10 Afzelius, B.A.; Gargani, G.; Romano, C.: Abnormal length of cilia as a possible cause of defective mucociliary clearance. Eur. J. resp. Dis. *66:* 173–180 (1985).

11 Ahmed, T.; Januszkiewicz, A.J.; Lauda, J.F.; Brown, A.; Chapman, G.A.; Kenny, P.J.; Finn, R.D.; Bondick, J.; Sackner, M.A.: Effect of local radioactivity on tracheal mucous velocity of sheep. Am. Rev. resp. Dis. *120:* 567–575 (1979).

12 Ahonen, A.; Valavirta, K.: Ultrastructure of cilia in pulmonary tuberculosis. Eur. J. resp. Dis. *64:* suppl. 128, pp. 460–463 (1983).

13 Ailsby, R.L.; Ghardially, F.N.: Atypical cilia in human bronchial mucosa. J. Path. *109:* 75–78 (1973).

14 Akkoclu, G.; Konietzko N.: Einfluss von Ipratropiumbromid auf die Ziliarkinetik menschlicher Nasenmukosa in vitro. Atemwegs-Lungenkr. *11:* 527–530 (1985).

15 Albegger, K.W.: Zilienveränderungen bei chronischer Sinusitis maxillaris. Eine raster- und transmissionselektronmikroskopische Untersuchung. Laryng. Rhinol. Otol. *57:* 395–405 (1978).

16 Albert, R.E.; Arnett, L.C.: Clearance of radioactive dust from the lung. Arch. Ind. Hlth *12:* 99–105 (1955).

17 Albertsson, M.; Mercke, C.; Hakansson, C.H.; von Mecklenburg, C.: Scanning elec-

tron microscopy and transmission electron microscopy of the ciliated cells of the trachea of the rabbit treated with misonidazol alone and in combination with ionizing radiation. Radiotherapy Oncology *3:* 47–60 (1985).

18 Alexander, F.W.: Micropathology of radiation reaction in the larynx. Ann. Otol. *72:* 831–841 (1963).

19 Amabile, G.; Bordiga, E.; Sardi, G.: Taratura del test della saccarina per la valutazione della clearance mucociliare delle fosse nasali. Otorhinolaryngologica *34:* 469–472 (1984).

20 Andersen, H.C.; Solgaard, J.; Andersen, I.: Nasal cancer and nasal mucus transport rates in woodworkers. Acta oto-lar. *82:* 263–265 (1976).

21 Andersen, I.; Camner, P.; Jensen, P.L.; Philipson, K.; Proctor, D.F.: Nasal clearance in monozygotic twins. Am. Rev. resp. Dis. *110:* 301 (1974).

22 Andersen, I.; Proctor, D.F.: The fate and effects of inhaled materials; in Proctor, Andersen, The nose (Elsevier, Amsterdam 1982).

23 Andreasson, L.; Björlin, G.; Hocherman, M.; Korsgaard, R.; Trell, E.: Laryngeal cancer, aryl hydrocarbon hydroxylase inducibility and smoking. ORL *49:* 187–192 (1987).

24 Antweiler, H.: Über die Funktion des Flimmerepithels der Luftwege, insbesondere unter Staubbelastung. Beiträge zur Silikoseforschung, Sonderband, Grundfragen der Silikoseforschung (Bergbau-Berufsgenossenschaft, Bochum 1958).

25 Ardan, G.M.; Kemp, F.: The mechanisms of the larynx. Part I: The movements of the arytenoid and cricoid cartilages. Brit. J. Radiol. *39:* 641–654 (1966).

26 Armengot, M.; Marco, J.: Variaciones del aclariamento mucociliar nasal en sujetos normales y con diversas patologicas nasales. Acta otolar. Español. *37:* 319–324 (1986).

27 van As, A.; Betty, J.: Postnatal adaption of ciliary function to temperature and pH. Am. Rev. resp. Dis. *132:* suppl. 4, A 73 (1986).

28 van der Baan, S.; Veerman, A.J.P.; Wulffraat, N.; Bezemer, P.D.; Feenstra, L.: Primary ciliary dyskinesia: ciliary activity. Acta oto-lar. *102:* 274–281 (1986).

29 Baetjer, A.M.; Bates, L.M.: Measurement of ciliary activity in the intact trachea. Am. Rev. resp. Dis. *93:* suppl., pp. 79–82 (1966).

30 Baldetorp, L.; Huberman, D.; Hakansson, C.H.; Toremalm, N.G.: Effects of ionizing radiation on the activity of the ciliated epithelium of the trachea. Acta radiol. (Ther.) *15:* 225–232 (1976).

31 Baldetorp, L.; von Mecklenburg, C.; Hakansson, C.H.: Ultrastructural alterations in ciliary cells exposed to ionizing radiation. Cell. Tiss. Res. *180:* 421–431 (1977).

32 Ballenger, J.J.; Dawson, F.W.; DeRuyter, M.G.; Harding, H.B.: Effects of nicotine on ciliary activity in vitro. Ann. Otol., St Louis *74:* 303 (1965).

33 Ballenger, J.J.; Harding, H.B.; Dawson, F.W.; DeRuyter, M.G.; Moore, J.A.: Cultural methods for measuring ciliary activity. Am. Rev. resp. Dis. *93:* 61–66 (1966).

34 Ballenger, J.J.: Some effects of formaldehyde on the upper respiratory tract. Laryngoscope, St Louis *94:* 1411–1413 (1984).

35 Bang, F.B.; Bang, B.G.; Foard, M.A.: Responses of upper respiratory mucosa to drugs and viral infection. Am. Rev. resp. Dis. *93:* 142–149 (1966).

36 Barclay, A.E.; Franklin, K.J.: The rate of excretion of india ink injected into the lungs. J. Physiol., London *90:* 482–488 (1937).

37   Bartholmé, W.; Karduck, A.: 10-Jahres-Erfahrung mit der Transkonioskopie in der laryngologischen Diagnostik. HNO 25: 273–275 (1977).

38   Baum, G.L.; Roth, Y.; Teichtahl, H.; Aharonson, E.; Priel, Z.: Ciliary beat frequency of respiratory mucosal cells: comparison of nasal and tracheal sampling sites. Am. Rev. resp. Dis. 125: Annual Meeting, suppl. 4/82, part 2, 244 (1982).

39   Becker, B.; Morgenroth, K.; Reinhardt, D.; Irlich, G.: The dyskinetic cilia syndrome in childhood. Modifications of ultrastructural patterns. Respiration 46: 180–186 (1984).

40   Beigel, A.; Steffens-Knutzen, R.; Tillmann, B.; Müller-Buchholz, W.: Trachealtransplantation, Vergleich von Reaktionen gegen vitale und unterschiedlich konservierte Trachealtransplantate bei Ratteninzuchtstämmen. Archs Oto-Rhino-Lar., suppl. 2, p. 244 (1984).

41   Bernfeld, P.; Keller, T.F.; Homburger, F.: Ciliary activity in mucus-free and mucus-covered tissues. Am. Rev. resp. Dis. 93: suppl., pp. 74–78 (1966).

42   Bertrand, B.; Degen, A.: Ciliary abnormalities in children (hockey-stick cilia). Study by scanning electron microscope. Report on three pediatric cases. Acta oto-rhinolar. belg. 38: 337–344 (1984).

43   Bertrand, B.: Endoscopic method for the measurement of the mucociliary clearance of maxillary sinus; in Clement, Recent advances in ENT-endoscopy (Scientific Society for Medical Information, Gent 1985).

44   Biondi, S.; Biondi-Zappala, M.: Surface of laryngeal mucosa seen through the scanning electron microscope. Folia phoniat. 26: 241–248 (1974).

45   Birch, L.; Elbrond, O.: Mucociliary function in the nasal cavity of children and adolescents with cholesteatoma. Clin. Otolaryngol. 11: 15–19 (1986).

46   Birnmeyer, G.: Der Verlauf des Inspirationsstromes im Kehlkopf. Arch. Ohr.-Nas. KehlkHeilk. 174: 369–374 (1959).

47   Birnmeyer, G.: Inhalationsnoxen und ortsfremdes Plattenepithel im Larynx. Arch. Gewerbepathol. Gewerbehyg. 17: 294–315 (1959).

48   Birzle, H.: Röntgenographische Darstellung der Flimmerbewegung des Trachealepithels; Versuche an isolierten Luftröhren von Schlachttieren. Fortschr. Röntgenstr. 84: 566–670 (1956).

49   Blum, H.C.; Petro, W.; Rutayangwa, E.; Konietzko, N.: In vitro cholinergic stimulation of human cilia. 4. Kongress der Europäischen Gesellschaft für Pulmologie, Stresa 1985.

50   Breuninger, H.: Über das physikalisch-chemische Verhalten des Nasenschleimes. Arch. Ohr.-Nas. KehlkHeilk. 184: 133–138 (1964).

51   Bridger, G.P.; Proctor, D.F.: Laryngeal mucociliary clearance. Ann. Otol., St Louis 80: 445–449 (1971).

52   Bridger, G.P.; Proctor, D.F.: Mucociliary function in the dog's larynx and trachea. Laryngoscope, St Louis 82: 218–224 (1972).

53   Brinkman, D.: Discussion to Rhodin, J.: Ultrastructure and function of human tracheal mucosa. Am. Rev. resp. Dis. 93: suppl. 60 (1966).

54   Brokaw, C.J.: Mechanics and energetics of cilia. Am. Rev. resp. Dis. 93: suppl., pp. 32–40 (1966).

55   Brondeel, L.; Sönstabö, R.; Clement, P.; van Ryckeghem, W.; van den Broek, M.: Value of the Tc^{99m} particle test and the saccharine test in mucociliary examinations. Rhinology 21: 135–142 (1983).

56 Brown, D.T.; Potsic, W.P.; Marsh, R.R.; Lift, M.: Drugs affecting clearance of middle ear secretions: a perspective for the management of otitis media with effusion. Ann. Otol. *94:* suppl., p. 117 (1985).

57 Bryan, W.T.K.; Bryan, M.P.; Smith, C.A.: Human ciliated epithelial cells in nasal secretions. Ann. Otol. *37:* 474–486 (1964).

58 Buratti, C.: Aspetti morfologici dei tessuti laringei non tumorali colpiti dal fascio radiante in corso di terapia con gli elettroni accelerati del betatrone per carcinoma. Ann. Laryng. *67:* 809–827 (1969).

59 Burgersdijk, F.J.A.; de Groot, J.C.M.J.; Graamans, K.; Rademakers, L.H.P.M.: Testing ciliary activity in patients with chronic and recurrent infection of the upper airways: experience in 68 cases. Laryngoscope, St Louis *96:* 1029–1033 (1986).

60 Burian, K.: Über die Restitutionsfähigkeit des Flimmerepithels der Nase nach totaler Zerstörung des Epithels. Z. Lar. Rhinol. Otol. *39:* 387–395 (1960).

61 Burian, K.; Stockinger, L.: Elektronenmikroskopische Untersuchungen an der Nasenschleimhaut. I. Das Flimmerepithel nach lokalen Schädigungen. Acta oto-lar. *56:* 376–389 (1963).

62 Burkert, Th.: Untersuchungen des kultivierten Flimmerepithels des oberen Respirationstraktes im Durchlichtmikroskop. Österreichischer HNO-Kongress/Donaustaatensymposium 1984 und persönliche Mitteilungen.

63 Byloos, J.; Ramet, J.; Clement, P.A.R.; Dehaen, F.: Transmissionselektronenmikroskopische Untersuchungen der Cilien. Acta oto-rhino-lar. belg. *38:* 391–400 (1984).

64 Camner, P.; Philipson, K.; Friberg, L.; Holma, B.; Larsson, B.; Svedbergh, J.: Human tracheobronchial clearance studies. Arch. envir. Hlth *22:* 444–449 (1971).

65 Camner, P.; Philipson, K.; Friberg, L.: Tracheobronchial clearance in twins. Arch. envir. Hlth *24:* 82–87 (1972).

66 Camner, P.; Strandberg, K.; Philipson, K.: Increased mucociliary transport by adrenergic stimulation. Arch. envir. Hlth *31:* 79–82 (1976).

67 Carson, S.; Goldhamer, R.; Carpenter, R.: Mucus transport in the respiratory tract. Am. Rev. resp. Dis. *93:* suppl., pp. 86–92 (1966).

68 Carson, J.L.; Collier, A.M.; Knowles, M.R.; Boucher, R.C.; Rose, J.G.: Morphometric aspects of ciliary distribution and ciliogenesis in human nasal epithelium. Proc. natn. Acad. Sci. USA *78:* 6996–6999 (1981).

69 Carson, J.L.; Collier, A.M.; Shih-Chin, S.H.: Acquired ciliary defects in nasal epithelium of children with acute viral upper respiratory infections. New Engl. J. Med. *312:* 463–468 (1985).

70 Cavaliere, F.; Carducci, P.; Schiavello, R.; Masieri, S.; Gobbi, L.; Passali, D.: Meccanismo della depressione mucociliare indotta dall'alotano: osservazione a favore di un'azione diretta sull'epitelio in vivo. Riv. ital. ORL Audiol. Foniat. *5:* 105–106 (1985).

71 Centanni, S.; Camporesi, E.; Allegra, L.: Atropine effect on ciliary beat frequency of respiratory epithelium. 4. Kongress der Europäischen Gesellschaft für Pulmologie, Stresa, 1985.

72 Charton, J.; Rigaud, A.; Grateau, P.; Cudennec, Y.F.; Buffe, P.: L'immobilité ciliaire nasale et son retentissement otologique. Ann. Otol. Lar., Paris *102:* 91–95 (1985).

73 Chen, T.M.; Dulfano, M.J.: Mucus viscoelasticity and mucociliary transport rate. J. Lab. clin. Med. *91:* 423–431 (1978).

74   Chevance, L.G.; Lennon, J.F.; Renaud-Mornaut, J.: Etudes des rhythmes du batte-
      ment ciliaire. Acta oto-lar. *70:* 16–28 (1970).

75   Chladek, V.: Cytology of the nasal secretion with a special regard to the diagnosis of
      allergical phenomena. Acta oto-lar. *35:* 508–515 (1947).

76   Cohen, D.; Arai, S.F.; Brain, J.D.: Smoking impairs long-term dust clearance from
      the lung. Science *204:* 514–517 (1979).

77   Connolly, T.P.; Noujaim, A.A.; Paul Man, S.F.: Simultaneous canine tracheal trans-
      port of different particles. Am. Rev. resp. Dis. *118:* 965–968 (1978).

78   Corkey, D.W.B.; Levison, H.; Turner, J.A.P.: The immotile cilia syndrome. Am.
      Rev. resp. Dis. *124:* 544–548 (1981).

79   Corssen, G.; Allen, C.R.: Cultured human respiratory epithelium: its use in the
      comparison of the cytotoxic properties of local anaesthetics. Anesthesiology *21:*
      237–243 (1960).

80   Dalhamn, T.; Rylander, R.: Frequency of ciliary beat measured with a photosensi-
      tive cell. Nature *196:* 592–599 (1962).

81   Dalhamn, T.; Rylander, R.: Ciliastatic action of cigarette smoke. Arch. oto-lar. *81:*
      379 (1965).

82   Dalhamn, T.: Effect of cigarette smoke on ciliary activity. Am. Rev. resp. Dis. *93:*
      suppl., pp. 108–114 (1966).

83   Deitmer, J.W.: Evidence for two voltage-dependent calcium currents in the mem-
      brane of the ciliate stylonychia. J. Physiol., Lond. *355:* 137–159 (1984).

84   Deitmer, T.: A method for standardizing cytologic sampling for the estimation of
      nasal ciliary activity. Archs Oto-Rhino-Lar. *243:* 288–292 (1986).

85   Deitmer, T.: Der Einfluss der Strahlentherapie auf die Funktion des Flimmerepi-
      thels im Kehlkopf. Lar. Rhinol. Otol. *65:* 513–515 (1986).

86   Deitmer, T.: A modification of the saccharine test for nasal mucociliary clearance.
      Rhinology *24:* 237–240 (1986).

87   Deitmer, T.: Untersuchungen zur Methodik des vital-cytologischen Abstriches vom
      Flimmerepithel. Atemwegs-Lungenkr. *13:* 133–137 (1987).

88   Deitmer, T.; Erwig, H.: The influence of nasal obstruction on mucociliary transport.
      Rhinology *24:* 159–162 (1986).

89   Dentler, W.A.: Microtubule-membrane interactions in cilia and flagella. Int. Rev.
      Cytol. *72:* 1–47 (1981).

90   Dixon, W.E.; Inchley, O.: The cilioscribe, an instrument for recording the activity of
      cilia. J. Physiol. *32:* 395–400 (1905).

91   Dolowitz, D.A.; Dougherty, T.F.: A study of cilia and connective tissue in normal
      and hyperplastic nasal mucous membrane. Laryngoscope, St Louis *76:* 1380–1388
      (1966).

92   von den Donk, H.J.M.; Zuidema, J.; Merkus, F.W.H.M.: The influence of the pH
      and osmotic pressure upon tracheal ciliary beat frequency as determined with a new
      photo-electric registration device. Rhinology *18:* 93–104 (1980).

93   van den Donk, H.J.M.; Müller-Plantema, I.P.; Ziudema, J.; Merkus, F.W.H.M.: The
      effects of preservatives on the ciliary beat frequency of chicken embryo tracheas.
      Rhinology *18:* 119–133 (1980).

94   van den Donk, H.J.M.; van den Heuvel, A.G.M.; Zuidema, J.; Merkus, F.W.H.M.:
      The effects of nasal drops and their additives on human nasal, mucociliary clear-
      ance. Rhinology *20:* 127–137 (1982).

95 Douglas, R.G.; Alford, B.R.; Couch, R.B.: Atraumatic nasal biopsy for studies of respiratory virus infection in volunteers. Antimicrob. Agents Chemother. *8:* 340–343 (1969).

96 Doyle, W.J.; van Cauwenberge, P.B.: Relation between nasal patency and clearance. Rhinology *25:* 167–179 (1987).

97 Drettner, B.; Aust, R.: Pathophysiology of the paranasal sinuses. Acta oto-lar. *83:* 16–19 (1977).

98 Drettner, B.: The paranasal sinuses; in Proctor, Andersen, The nose (Elsevier, Amsterdam 1982).

99 Drucker, J.; Weisman, Z.; Sadé, J.: Tissue culture of human adult adenoids and of middle ear mucosa. Ann. Otol. *85:* 327–333 (1976).

100 Duchateau, G.S.M.J.E.; Graamans, K.; Zuidema, J.; Merkus, F.W.H.M.: Correlation between nasal ciliary beat frequency and mucus transport rate in volunteers. Laryngoscope *95:* 854–859 (1985).

101 Duchateau, G.S.M.J.E.; Zuidema, J.; Merkus F.W.H.M.: The in vitro and in vivo effect of a new non-halogenated corticosteroid – budesonide – aerosol on human ciliary epithelial function. Allergy *41:* 260–265 (1986).

102 Dudley, J.P.; Welch, M.J.; Stiehm, E.R.; Carney, J.M.; Sonderberg-Warner, M.: Scanning and transmission electron microscopy aspect of the nasal acilia syndrome. Laryngoscope, St Louis *92:* 297–299 (1982).

103 Dudley, J.P.; Cherry, J.D.; Eisner, L.: Scanning electron microscopy examination of nonbeating cilia. Ann. Otol. *91:* 612–614 (1982).

104 Eavey, R.D.; Nadol, J.B.; Holmes, L.B.; Laird, N.M.; Lapey, A.; Joseph, M.P.; Strome, M.: Karatagener's syndrome, a blinded controlled study of cilia ultrastructure. Archs Oto-Rhino-Lar. *112:* 646–650 (1986).

105 Eichner, H.: Eine neue Methode zur Gewinnung von Nasensekret und erste Untersuchungen zur Eiweisszusammensetzung des Nasensekretes mittels Diskelektrophorese. Lar. Rhinol. Otol. *53:* 269–275 (1979).

106 Elbrond, O.; Larsen, E.: Mucociliary function of the eustachian tube. Arch. Otolar. *102:* 539–541 (1976).

107 El-Hifnawi, H.; El-Hifnawi, E.: Light and electron microscopical studies of the anatomical and functional distribution of glands in human vocal cords. Archs Oto-Rhino-Lar. *240:* 277–285 (1984).

108 Eliasson, R.; Mossberg, B.; Camner, P.; Afzelius, B.A.: The immotile cilia syndrome. A congenital ciliary abnormality as an etiologic factor in chronic airway infections and male sterility. New Engl. J. Med. *297:* 1–6 (1977).

109 Elverland, H.H.: Kartagener's syndrome – a reappraisal. Acta oto-lar., suppl. 360, pp. 129–130 (1979).

110 Elwany, S.: Delayed ultrastructural radiation induced changes in the human mesotympanic middle ear mucosa. J. Lar. Otol. *99:* 343–353 (1985).

111 Elwany, S.; Bumstedt, R.: Ultrastructural observations on vasomotor rhinitis. ORL *49:* 199–205 (1987).

112 Engelmann, Th.W.: Flimmeruhr und Flimmermühle. Zwei Apparate zum Registrieren der Flimmerbewegung. Pflügers Arch. Ges. Physiol. *15:* 494–510 (1877).

113 Engström, H.: The structure of tracheal cilia. Acta oto-lar. *39:* 360–366 (1951).

114 Ernestson, S.; Afzelius, B.A.; Mossberg, B.: Otologic manifestations of the immotile-cilia syndrome. Acta oto-lar. *97:* 83–92 (1984).

115 Escudier, E.; Bernaudin, J.F.; Bernaudin, Ph.; Reinert, Ph.; Canet, J.; Boncherat, M.; Peynegre, R.: Etude stroboscopique de la fréquence des battements des cils de la muqueuse respiratoire. Ann. Oto-Lar., Paris *101:* 150–152 (1984).

116 de Espana, R.; Franch, M.; Garcia, A.; Pavia, J.: Measurement of nasal mucociliary transport rate in man. Rhinology *24:* 241–247 (1986).

117 Ewert, G.: On the mucus flow rate in the human nose. Acta oto-lar., suppl. 200, pp. 1–62 (1965).

118 Ewert, G.; Martensson, B.: Mucus flow in the subglottic region studied by transconioscopy. Acta oto-lar., suppl. 224, pp. 515–517 (1967).

119 Falser, N.: Kinozilienanomalien beim Kartagener-Syndrom. Lar. Rhinol. Otol. *62:* 128–132 (1983).

120 Fawcett, D.W.; Porter, K.R.: A study of the fine structure of ciliated epithelium. J. Morph. *94:* 221–264 (1954).

121 Fazio, F.; Lafortuna, C.: Effect of inhaled salbutamol on mucociliary clearance in patients with chronic bronchitis. Chest *80:* suppl., pp. 827–830 (1981).

122 Felix, H.; ElSayed, H.; Nauer, R.: Funktionelle Untersuchungen am Flimmerepithel der Eustachischen Tube beim Menschen. Zentbl. Hals-Nasen-Ohrenheilk. *133:* 636 (1986).

123 Finnström, O.; Ödkvist, L.; Afzelius, B.A.: The immotile cilia syndrome in a newborn infant. Int. J. pediat. Otorhinolaryngol. *2:* 33–37 (1980).

124 Fontoillet, C.; Terrier, G.: Abnormalities of cilia and chronic sinusitis. Rhinology *25:* 57–62 (1987).

125 Forrest, J.B.; Rossman, C.M.; Newhouse, M.T.; Ruffin, R.: Activation of nasal cilia in immotile cilia syndrome. Am. Rev. resp. Dis. *120:* 511–515 (1979).

126 Foster, W.M.; Langenback, E.; Bergofsky, E.H.: Measurement of tracheal and bronchial mucus velocities in man: relation to lung clearance. J. appl. Physiol. *48:* 965–971 (1980).

127 Foster, W.M.; Costa, D.L.; Langenback, E.G.: Ozone exposure alters tracheobronchial mucociliary function in man. Am. Rev. resp. Dis. *132:* suppl. 4, A 216 (1986).

128 Fox, B.; Bull, T.B.; Arden, G.B.: Variations in the ultrastructure of human nasal cilia including abnormalities found in retinitis pigmentosa. J. clin. Pathol. *33:* 327–335 (1980).

129 Fox, B.; Bull, T.B.; Makey, A.R.; Rawbone, R.: The significance of ultrastructural abnormalities of human cilia. Chest *80:* suppl., pp. 796–799 (1981).

130 Frenckner, P.: The effect of roentgen and radium radiation upon the action of cilia within the respiratory tract. Acta oto-lar. *27:* 297–309 (1939).

131 Friedman, I.; Bird, E.S.: Ciliary structure, ciliogenesis, microvilli. Laryngoscope, St Louis *91:* 1852–1868 (1971).

132 Friedman, M.; Stott, F.D.; Poole, D.O.; Dougherty, R.; Chapman, G.A.; Watson, H.; Sackner, M.A.: A new roentgenographic method for estimating mucous velocity in airways. Am. Rev. resp. Dis. *155:* 67–75 (1977).

133 Fujiwara, K.; Hakansson, H.C.; Toremalm, N.G.: Influence of ionizing radiation on ciliary cell activity in the respiratory tract. Acta radiol. (Ther.) *11:* 513–520 (1972).

134 Fujiwara, K.; Hakansson, C.H.; Toremalm, N.G.: Studies on the physiology of the trachea. VI. Interaction between ciliary beat frequency and transport of secretions. Ann. Otol. *81:* 212–217 (1972).

135 Gelman, R.A.; Meyer, F.A.: Mucociliary transference rate and mucus viscoelasticity. Dependence on dynamic storage and loss modulus. Am. Rev. resp. Dis. *120:* 553–557 (1979).

136 George, R.J.D.; Moore-Gillon, V.; Geddes, D.M.: High frequency oscillations improve nasal mucociliary clearance. Lancet *ii:* 10–12 (1984).

137 Gibbons, I.R.; Rowe, A.J.: Dynein: a protein with adenosine triphosphatase activity from cilia. Science *149:* 424–426 (1965).

138 Ginzel, A.; Illum, P.: Nasal mucociliary clearance in patients with septal deviation. Rhinology *18:* 177–181 (1980).

139 Giordano, A.; Holsclaw, D.S.: Tracheal resection and mucociliary clearance. Ann. Otol. *85:* 631–639 (1976).

140 Giordano, A.; Shih, Ch.K.; Holsclaw, D.S.; Khan, M.A.; Litt, M.: Mucus clearance: in vivo canine tracheal vs. in vitro bullfrog palate studies. J. appl. Physiol. *42:* 761–766 (1977).

141 Giordano, A.; Holsclaw, D.; Litt, M.: Mucus rheology and mucociliary clearance: normal physiologic state. Am. Rev. resp. Dis. *118:* 245–250 (1978).

142 Goldhaber, G.; Back, A.: Studies on radiosensitivity of animal cell in vitro. I. Radiosensitivity of muscular and ciliary movement. Proc. Soc. exp. Biol. Med. *48:* 150–151 (1941).

143 Golhar, S.: Nasal mucus clearance. J. Lar. Otol. *100:* 533–538 (1986).

144 Gosselin, R.E.: Physiologic regulators of ciliary motion. Am. Rev. resp. Dis. *93:* suppl., pp. 41–59 (1966).

145 Grammatica, L.; Latorre, F.; Barbara, M.: Il trasporto muco-ciliare e la poliposo nasale. Otorinolaryngologica *35:* 421–423 (1985).

146 Gray, J.: Ciliary movement (Cambridge University Press, Cambridge 1928).

147 Gray, J.: The mechanisms of ciliary movement. Photographic and stroboscopic analysis of ciliary movement. Proc. R. Soc. Biol. *107:* 313–318 (1930).

148 Greenstone, M.; Cooper, P.; Warner, J.; Cole, P.J.: Effect of acute antigenic challenge on nasal ciliary beat frequency. Eur. J. resp. Dis. *64:* suppl. 128, pp. 449–450 (1983).

149 Greenstone, M.; Stanley, P.; MacWilliam, L.; Dewar, A.; Cox, T.; Mackay, I.S.; Cole, P.J.: Mucociliary function and ciliary ultrastructure in patients presenting with rhinitis to Brompton Hospital Nose Clinic. Eur. J. resp. Dis. *64:* suppl. 128, pp. 457–459 (1983).

150 Greenstone, M.; Stanley, P.; Cole, P.; Mackay, I.: Upper airway manifestations of primary ciliary dyskinesia. J. Lar. Otol. *99:* 985–991 (1985).

151 Griffith, D.E.; Holden, W.E.; Morris, J.F.; Min, L.K.; Krishnamurthy, G.T.: Effects of common therapeutic concentrations of oxygen on lung clearance of ^{99m}Tc-DTPA and bronchoalveolar lavage albumin concentration. Am. Rev. resp. Dis. *134:* 233–237 (1966).

152 Grossan, M.: The saccharine test of nasal mucociliary function. Eye Ear Nose Throat Mon. *54:* 415–417 (1975).

153 Gruenauer, L.M.; Grotberg, J.B.; Miller, I.F.; Yeates, D.B.: Fluid transport by high frequency asymmetric air flow. Am. Rev. resp. Dis. *132:* suppl. 4, A 74 (1986).

154 Güney, E.; Tanyeri, Y.; Kandemir, B.; Yalcin, S.: The effect of wood dust on the nasal cavity and paranasal sinuses. Rhinology *25:* 273–277 (1987).

155 Gunnarson, M.; Hybbinette, J.C.; Mercke, U.: Mucolytic agents and mucociliary activity. Rhinology *22:* 223–231 (1984).

156 Hachenberg, T.; Wendt, M.; Deitmer, T.; Lawin, P.: Viscoelasticity of tracheobronchial secretions in high-frequency ventilation. Crit. Care Med. *15:* 95–98 (1987).

157 Hakansson, C.H.; Toremalm, N.G.: Studies on the physiology of the trachea. I. Ciliary activity indirectly recorded by a new 'light beam reflex' method. Ann. Otol. *74:* 954–969 (1965).

158 Hakansson, C.H.; Toremalm, N.G.: Studies on the physiology of the trachea. III. Electrical activity of the ciliary cell layer. Ann. Otol. *75:* 1007–1018 (1966).

159 Hakansson, C.H.; Toremalm, N.G.: Studies on the physiology of the trachea. II. Electrical potential gradients within the tracheal wall. Ann. Otol. *75:* 33–47 (1966).

160 Hakansson, C.H.; Toremalm, N.G.: Studies on the physiology of the trachea. IV. Electrical and mechanical activity of the smooth muscles. Ann. Otol. *76:* 873–884 (1967).

161 Hakansson, C.H.; Toremalm, N.G.: Studies on the physiology of the trachea. V. Histology and mechanical activity of the smooth muscles. Ann. Otol. *77:* 255–263 (1968).

162 Hakansson, C.H.; Toremalm, N.G.: A method for determining the viscoelasticity of tracheobronchial secretions. Am. Rev. resp. Dis. *102:* 47–53 (1970).

163 Hakansson, C.H.; Toremalm, N.G.: Ciliary activity recorded by TV-monitor and phototube. Acta oto-lar. *71:* 508–510 (1971).

164 Hansell, M.M.; Moretti, R.L.: Ultrastructure of the mouse tracheal epithelium. J. Morph. *128:* 159–170 (1969).

165 Harmsen, A.G.; Muggenburg, B.A.; Bice, D.E.: The role of lung phagocytes in the clearance of particles by the mucociliary apparatus. Am. Rev. resp. Dis. *132:* suppl. 4, A 48 (1986).

166 Harris, C.C.; Kaufman, D.G.; Jackson, F.; Smith, J.M.; Dedick, P.; Saffioti, U.: Atypical cilia in the tracheobronchial epithelium of the hamster during respiratory carcinogenesis. J. Pathol. *114:* 17–19 (1974).

167 Hastie, A.T.: Inhibition of mammalian ciliary activity by formaldehyde. Am. Rev. resp. Dis. *132:* suppl. 4, A 84 (1986).

168 de Heide, A.: Anatome, mytuli, belgica mossel (Amsterdam 1684).

169 Heine, L.H.: The effect of radiation upon ciliated epithelium. Ann. Otol. *45:* 60 (1936).

170 Hermens, W.A.J.J.; Schüssler van Hees, M.T.I.W.; Merkus, F.W.H.M.: The in vitro effect of morphine, fentanyl, and sufentanil on ciliary beat frequency of human nasal epithelial tissue. Acta pharm. technol. *33:* 88–90 (1987).

171 Herrmann, A.: Zur Physiologie und Pathologie der Schleimhautfunktion in Luftröhre und Bronchien und ihre Bedeutung für die Klinik. Zentbl. Hals-Nasen-Ohrenheilk. *36:* 279–287 (1934).

172 Hers, J.F.Ph.: Disturbances of the ciliated epithelium due to influenza virus. Am. Rev. resp. Dis. *93:* suppl., pp. 162–171 (1966).

173 Herzon, F.S.; Murphy, S.: Normal ciliary ultrastructure in children with Kartagener's syndrome. Ann. Otol. *89:* 81–83 (1980).

174 Herzon, F.S.: Upper respiratory tract ciliary ultrastructural pathology. Ann. Otol., suppl. 83, pp. 1–12 (1981).

175 Herzon, F.S.: Nasal ciliary structural pathology. Laryngoscope, St Louis 63–67 (1983).

176 Hesse, H.; Kasparek, R.; Mizera, W.; Unterholzner, Ch.; Konietzko, N.: Influence of reproterol on ciliary beat frequency of human bronchial epithelium in vitro. Arzneimittel-Forsch. *31:* 716–718 (1981).

177 Heyder, J.: Mechanisms of aerosol particle deposition. Chest *80:* suppl., pp. 820–823 (1981).

178 Hilding, A.C.: The common cold. Arch. Otolar. *12:* 133 (1930).

179 Hilding, A.C.: The role of ciliary action in production of pulmonary atelectasis vaccum in the paranasal sinuses and in otitis media. Ann. Otol. *52:* 816–834 (1952).

180 Hilding, A.C.: Ciliary streaming through the larynx and distribution of laryngeal epithelium. Laryngoscope, St Louis *66:* 1362–1363 (1956).

181 Hilding, A.C.: On cigarette smoking, bronchial carcinoma and ciliary action. II. Experimental study on the filtering action of cows lungs, the disposition of tar in the bronchial tree and removal by ciliary action. New Engl. J. Med. *254:* 1155–1158 (1956).

182 Hilding, A.C.: On cigarette smoking, bronchial carcinoma and ciliary action. IV. Ciliary streaming through the larynx and distribution of laryngeal epithelium. Ann. Otol., St. Louis *56:* 736–746 (1956).

183 Hilding, A.C.: Ciliary streaming in the bronchial tree and the time element in carcinogenesis. New Engl. J. Med. *256:* 634–640 (1957).

184 Hilding, A.C.: Ciliary streaming through the larynx and trachea. J. thorac. Surg. *37:* 108–117 (1959).

185 Hilding, A.C.: Time-lapse relation to changes in the respiratory epithelium after minimal trauma. Acta oto-lar. *57:* 352–367 (1963).

186 Hilding, A.C.: Perspective and history of investigation of cilia in human disease. Am. Rev. resp. Dis. *93:* suppl., pp. 178–179 (1966).

187 Hilding. D.A.; Hilding, A.C.: Ultrastructure of tracheal cilia and cells during regeneration. Ann. Otol. *75:* 281–294 (1966).

188 Hills, B.A.: Analysis of eustachian surfactant and its function as a release agent. Archs Otolar. *110:* 3–9 (1984).

189 Hingley, S.T.; Hastie, A.T.; Higgins, M.L.; Kueppers, F.: Effect of pseudomonad proteases on mammalian ciliary activity. Am. Rev. resp. Dis. *132:* suppl. 4, A 73 (1986).

190 Hiramoto, Y.: Mechanics of ciliary movement; in Sleigh, Cilia and flagella (Academic Press, London 1974).

191 Hisamatsu, K.-J.; Yamauchi, Y.; Uchida, M.; Murakami, Y.: Promotive effect of lysozyme on the ciliary activity of the human nasal mucosa. Acta Otolar. *101:* 290–294 (1986).

192 Holmberg, K.; Pipkorn, U.: Mucociliary transport in the human nose. Effect of topical glucocorticoid treatment. Rhinology *23:* 181–185 (1985).

193 Honjo, I.: Clearance function of the eustachian tube. Ann. Otol. *94:* suppl. 120, pp. 29–30 (1985).

194 Hoorn, B.; Tyrell, D.A.J.: Effects of some viruses on ciliated cells. Am. Rev. resp. Dis. *93:* suppl., pp. 157–161 (1966).

195 Hybbinette, J.Ch.; Mercke, U.: A method for evaluating the effect of pharmacological substance in mucociliary activity in vivo. Acta oto-lar. *93:* 151–159 (1982).

196 Hybbinette, J.Ch.; Mercke, U.: Effects of the parasympathomimetic drug metacholine and its antagonist atropine on mucociliary activity. Acta oto-lar. *93:* 465–473 (1982).

197 Hybbinette, J.Ch.; Mercke, U.: Effects of sympathomimetic agonists and antagonists on mucociliary activity. Acta oto-lar. *94:* 121–130 (1982).

198 Iravani, J.: Flimmerbewegungen in den intrapulmonalen Luftwegen der Ratte. Pflügers Arch. ges. Physiol. *297:* 221–237 (1967).

199 Iravani, J.; van As, A.: Mucus transport in the tracheobronchial tree of normal and bronchitic rats. J. Pathol. *106:* 81–93 (1972).

200 Iravani, J.; Norris Melville, G.: Mucociliary activity in the respiratory tract as influenced by postaglandin E_1. Respiration *32:* 305–315 (1975).

201 Jafek, B.W.: Ultrastructure of human nasal mucosa. Laryngoscope, St Louis *93:* 1576–1599 (1983).

202 Jahnke, V.; Theopold, H.M.: Feinstruktur der Nasenschleimhaut bei Mucoviszidose unter besonderer Berücksichtigung der Polyposis. Lar. Rhinol. Otol. *56:* 773–781 (1977).

203 Jahnke, V.: Electron microscopy in rhinology. Rhinology *23:* 173–179 (1985).

204 Jahresdörfer, R.; Feldman, P.S.; Rubel, E.W.; Guerrant, J.L.; Eggelston, P.A.; Selden, R.F.: Otitis media and the immotile cilia syndrome. Laryngoscope, St Louis *89:* 769–778 (1979).

205 Jakse, R.; Popper, H.: Histologische Aspekte zur Diagnostik and Pathogenese des Kartagener Syndromes. Aktuelles in der ORL 1982, Österreich. HNO-Kongress, Bad Kleinkirchheim (Thieme, Stuttgart 1983).

206 Jakubikova, J.; Kapellerova, A.: Veränderungen des mucociliaren Transportes bei Kindern. Csl. otolar. *34:* 282–285 (1985).

207 Jakus, M.A.; Hall, C.E.: Electron microscope observations of trichocysts and cilia of paramecium. Biol. Bull. *91:* 131–146 (1946).

208 Jelinek, R.: Die Ausbreitung des Platten- und Flimmerepithels im Kehlkopf. Z. Lar. Rhinol. Otol. *45:* 1–5 (1966).

209 Johnson, N.; Villalon, M.; Verdugo, P.: Stereospecificity of the ATP-receptor in respiratory ciliated cells. Am. Rev. resp. Dis. *132:* suppl. 4, A 73 (1986).

210 Johnson, A.P.; Inzana, T.J.: Loss of ciliary activity in organ cultures of rat trachea treated with lipooligosaccharide from haemophilus influenzae. J. med. Microbiol. *22:* 265–268 (1986).

211 Juraske, P.; Arnold, W.; Wetzstein, R.: Oberflächenstruktur des normalen, präcancerösen und carcinomatösen Stimmbandepithels im Rasterelektronenmikroskop. Arch. Ohr-Nasen-KehlkHeilk. *210:* 243 (1975).

212 Kärja, J.; Nuutinen, J.; Karjaleinen, P.: Radioisotopic method for measurement of nasal mucociliary activity. Archs Otolar. *108:* 99–101 (1982).

213 Kärja, J.; Nuutinen, J.: Immotile cilia syndrome in children. Int. J. pediat. Otorhinolar. *5:* 275–279 (1983).

214 Karlsson, G.; Hansson, H.A.; Petruson, B.; Björkander, J.: The nasal mucosa in immunodeficiency. Acta oto-lar. *100:* 456–469 (1985).

215 Kawabata, J.; Paparella, M.: Atypical cilia in normal human and guinea pig middle ear mucosa. Acta oto-lar. *67:* 511–515 (1969).

216 Kaya, S.; Ercan, M.T.; Laleli, Y.: Measurement of nasal mucociliary activity in man with 99^mTc-labelled resin particles. Archs Oto-Rhino-Lar. *239:* 267–272 (1984).

217 Kensler, C.J.; Battista, S.P.: Chemical and physical factors affecting mammalian ciliary activity. Am. Rev. resp. Dis. *93:* suppl., pp. 93–102 (1966).

218 Kennedy, J.R.; Duckett, K.E.: The study of ciliary frequencies with an optical spectrum analysis system. Expl Cell Res. *135:* 47–56 (1981).

219 Kihara, S.; Ohashi, Y.; Maruoka, K.; Ikeoka, H.; Masutani, H.; Nakai, Y.: The ciliary activity of the middle ear lining in some pathological states. Auris nasus larynx *12:* suppl. 1, pp. 126–128 (1985).

220 Kilburn, K.H.; Salzano, J.V.: Foreword: Symposium on structure, function and measurement of respiratory cilia. Am. Rev. resp. Dis. *93:* suppl., p. 1 (1966).

221 King, M.; Gilboa, A.; Meyer, F.A.; Silberberg, A.: On the transport of mucus and its rheologic stimultans in ciliated systems. Am. Rev. resp. Dis. *110:* 740 (1974).

222 Kleinsasser, O.: Über die Histogenese und das Wachstum junger Kehlkopfkrebse. Z. Lar. Rhinol. Otol. *42:* 499–520 (1963).

223 Kleinsasser, O.: Bösartige Geschwülste des Kehlkopfes und des Hypopharynx; in Berendes, Link, Zöllner, Hals-Nasen-Ohrenheilkunde in Praxis und Klinik, Bd. 4/2 (Thieme, Stuttgart 1983).

224 Kleinsasser, O.: Tumoren des Kehlkopfes und Hypopharynx (Thieme, Stuttgart 1987).

225 Köhler, D.; Fischer, J.; Rühle, K.H.; Gaede, J.; Matthys, H.: Ziliarer und nichtziliarer Partikeltransport; in Rensch, Mukustransport (Dustri, München 1980).

226 Konietzko, N.: Die Bronchialwegsreinigung: Möglichkeiten ihrer Beeinflussung. Therapiewoche *26:* 8230–8243 (1976).

227 Konietzko, N.; Klopfer M.; Adam, W.E.; Matthys, H.: Die mukociliäre Klärfunktion der Lunge unter β-adrenerger Stimulation. Pneumologie *152:* 203–208 (1975).

228 Konietzko, N.; Nakhosteen, J.A.; Mizera, W.; Kasparek, R.; Hesse, H.: Ciliary beat frequency of biopsy samples taken from normal persons and patients with various lung diseases. Chest *80:* suppl., pp. 855–857 (1981).

229 Konietzko, N.; Kasparek, R.; Kellner, U.; Petro, J.: Die Wirkung von Bronchospasmolytika auf die Ciliarfrequenz in vitro. Prax. klin. Pneumol. *37:* 904–906 (1983).

230 Kotin, P.; Courington, D.; Falk, H.L.: Pathogenesis of cancer in ciliated mucus-secreting epithelium. Am. Rev. resp. Dis. *93:* suppl., pp. 115–124 (1966).

231 Kuschnir, H.: Direkte intratracheale Viskosimetrie von Tracheobronchialsekret. Lar. Rhinol. Otol. *61:* 93–94 (1982).

232 Laurenzi, G.A.; Guaneri, J.J.: A study of the mechanisms of pulmonary resistance to infection: the relationship of bacterial clearance to ciliary and alveolar macrophage function. Am. Rev. resp. Dis. *93:* suppl., pp. 134–141 (1966).

233 Lee, W.I.; Verdugo, P.: Laser light-scattering spectroscopy; a new application in study of ciliary activity. Biophys. J. *16:* 1115–1119 (1976).

234 Lee, W.I.; Verdugo, P.: Ciliary activity by laser light-scattering spectroscopy. Ann. biomed. Eng. *5:* 248–259 (1977).

235 Leitch, G.J.; Frid, L.H.; Phoenix, D.: The effect of ethanol on mucociliary clearance. Alcohol clin. exp. Res. *9:* 277–280 (1985).

236 Lenz, H.: Die Oberfläche der Nasenschleimhaut bei Rhinitis vasomotorica im Rasterelektronenmikroskop. Arch. Ohr-Nas.-Kehlkheilk. *202:* 353–359 (1972).

237 Lenz, H.: Die Oberflächenstruktur des nicht verhornenden Plattenepithel-Carcinoms des menschlichen Stimmbandes. Lar. Rhinol. *55:* 888–893 (1976).

238 Lierle, D.M.; Moore, P.M.: Further study of the effects of drugs on ciliary activity: a new method of observation in the living animal. Ann. Otol. *44:* 671–684 (1935).

239 Lindberg, S.; Mercke, U.: Bradykinin accelerates mucociliary activity in rabbit maxillary sinus. Acta oto-lar. *101:* 114–121 (1986).

240 Lindberg, S.; Mercke, U.; Uddman, R.: The morphological basis for the effect of

substance P on mucociliary activity in rabbit maxillary sinus. Acta oto-lar. *101:* 314–319 (1986).

241 Lindberg, S.; Hybbinette, J.Ch.; Mercke, U.: Effects of neuropeptides on mucociliary activity. Ann. Otol. Rhinol. Lar. *95:* 94–100 (1986).

242 Lindberg, S.; Mercke, U.: Antidromic nerve stimulation accelerates mucociliary activity in rabbit maxillary sinus. Acta oto-lar. *101:* 484–493 (1986).

243 Lindberg, S.; Dolata, J.; Mercke, U.: Nasal exposure to airway irritants triggers a mucociliary defence reflex in the rabbit maxillary sinus. Acta oto-lar. *104:* 552–560 (1987).

244 Lippmann, M.; Leikauf, G.; Spektor, D.; Schlesinger, R.B.; Albert, R.E.: The effect of irritant aerosols on mucus clearance from large and small conductive airways. Chest *80:* suppl., pp. 873–876 (1981).

245 Litt, M.D.: Physicochemical determinants of mucociliary flow. Chest *80:* suppl., pp. 846–849 (1981).

246 Lopez-Vidriero, M.T.: Airway mucus. Chest *80:* suppl., pp. 799–802 (1981).

247 Lopez-Vidriero, M.T.: Objective criteria for measuring ciliary beat frequency in vitro. Am. Rev. resp. Dis. *125:* Annual Meeting, suppl. 4/82, part 2, 244 (1982).

248 Lopez-Vidriero, M.T.; Jacobs, M.; Clarke, S.W.: The effect of isoprenaline on the ciliary activity of an in vitro preparation of rat trachea. Eur. J. Pharmacol. *112:* 429–432 (1985).

249 Lucas, A.M.: Coordination of ciliary movement, methods of study. J. Morph. *53:* 243–256 (1932).

250 Lucas, A.M.: Principles underlying ciliary activity in the respiratory tract. I. A method for direct observation of cilia in situ and its application. Archs Otolar. *18:* 516–524 (1933).

251 Lucas, A.M.; Douglas, L.C.: Principles underlying ciliary activity in the respiratory tract. II. A comparison of nasal clearance in man, monkey, and other mammals. Archs Otolar. *20:* 518–541 (1934).

252 Luk, C.K.; Dulfano, M.J.: Effect of pH, viscosity, and ionic strength on ciliary beating frequency of human bronchial explants. Am. Rev. resp. Dis. *125:* Annual Meeting, suppl. 4/82, part 2, 244 (1982).

253 Lundgren, J.; Olofson, J.; Hellquist, H.; Gröntoft, L.: Scanning electron microscopy of vocal cord hyperplasia, keratosis, papillomatosis, dysplasia and carcinoma. Acta oto-lar. *96:* 315–327 (1983).

254 Machemer, H.: Was bewegt einen Einzeller? Schriftenreihe der Westfälischen Wilhelms-Universität Münster, Heft 4 (Aschendorffsche Verlagsbuchhandl., Münster 1985).

255 Majima, Y.; Sakakura, Y.; Matsubara, T.; Hamaguchi, Y.; Hirata, K.; Takeuchi, K.; Miyoshi, Y.: Rheological properties of middle ear effusions from children with otitis media with effusion. Ann. Otol. *124:* suppl., pp. 1–4 (1986).

256 Majima, A.; Sakakura, Y.; Matsubara, Y.; Miyoshi, Y.: Possible mechanisms of reduction of nasal mucociliary clearance in chronic sinusitis. Clin. Otolaryngol. *11:* 55–60 (1986).

257 Manara, G.; Mira, E.: Modificazioni istologiche della laringe umana irradiata secondo diverse modalità tecnico-terapeutiche. Arch. ital. Otol. *79:* 595–635 (1968).

258 Marriott, Ch.: The viscoelastic nature of mucus secretions. Chest *80:* suppl., pp. 804–808 (1981).

259 Martensson, B.; Fluur, E.; Schiratzki, H.: Transconioscopy. A new method of laryngeal investigation. Acta oto-lar. *58:* 281–285 (1964).

260 Martin, R.; Litt, M.; Marriott, Ch.: The effect of mucolytic agents on the rheologic and transport properties of canine tracheal mucus. Am. Rev. resp. Dis. *121:* 495–500 (1980).

261 Martius, F.: Eine Methode zur absoluten Frequenzbestimmung der Flimmerbewegung auf stroboskopischem Wege. Arch. Anat. Physiol. *8:* 456–461 (1884).

262 Mass, M.J.; Lane, B.P.: Effect of chromates on ciliated cells of rat tracheal epithelium. Archs envir. Hlth *31:* 96–100 (1976).

263 Matthys, H.; Vastag, E.; Köhler, D.; Daikeler, G.; Fischer, J.: Mucociliary clearance in patients with chronic bronchitis and bronchial carcinoma. Respiration *44:* 329–337 (1983).

264 Maurizi, M.; Paludetti, G.; Todisco, T.; Almadori, G.; Ottaviani, F.; Zappone, C.: Ciliary ultrastructure and nasal mucociliary clearance in chronic and allergic rhinitis. Rhinology *22:* 233–240 (1984).

265 Maurizi, M.; Ottaviani, F.; Paludetti, G.; Almadori, G.; Zappone, C.: Adenoid hypertrophy and nasal mucociliary clearance in children. A morphological and functional study. Int. J. pediat. ORL *8:* 31–41 (1984).

266 Maurizi, M.; Ottaviani, F.; Paludetti, G.; Specra, A.; Almadori, G.: Choanal atresia: a surface and ultrastructural study of the nasal mucous membranes. Int. J. pediat. ORL *10:* 53–66 (1985).

267 Maurizi, M.; Paludetti, G.; Ottaviani, F.; Almadori, G.; Falcetti, S.: Mucociliary function and nasal resistance evaluation before and after adenoidectomy. Int. J. ped. ORL *11:* 295–300 (1986).

268 Maurizi, M.; Paludetti, G.; Almadori, G.; Ottaviani, F.; Todisco, T.: Mucociliary clearance and mucosal surface characteristics before and after total laryngectomy. Acta oto-lar. *102:* 136–145 (1986).

269 McCall, A.L.; Potsic, W.P.; Shih, C.K.; Litt, M.; Khan, M.A.: Physicochemical properties of human middle ear effusions (mucus) and their relation to ciliary transport. Laryngoscope, St Louis *88:* 729–737 (1978).

270 McLean, J.A.; Bacon, J.R.; Matheros, K.P.; Thrall, J.H.; Banas, J.M.; Hedden, J.; Bayne, N.K.: Distribution and clearance of radioactive aerosols on the nasal mucosa. Rhinology *22:* 65–75 (1984).

271 Mecklenburg, C. von; Mercke, U.; Hakansson, C.H.; Toremalm, N.G.: Morphological changes in ciliary cells due to heat exposure. Cell Tiss. Res. *148:* 45–56 (1974).

272 Meister, R.: Rauchgewohnheiten und Prävalenz broncho-pulmonaler Symptome in der Bevölkerung der Bundesrepublik; in Geisler, Rauchen und Atemwege (Verlag für angewandte Wissenschaften, München 1986).

273 Mercer, T.T.: Production of therapeutic aerosols. Chest *80:* suppl., pp. 813–818 (1981).

274 Mercke, U.; Hakansson, C.H.; Toremalm, N.G.: A method for standardized studies of mucociliary activity. Acta oto-lar. *78:* 118–123 (1974).

275 Mercke, U.: The influence of temperature on mucociliary activity. Acta oto-lar. *78:* 253–258 (1974).

276 Mercke, U.: The influence of varying air humidity on mucociliary activity. Acta oto-lar. *79:* 133–139 (1975).

277 Mercke, U.; Lindberg, S.; Dolata, J.: The role of neurokinin A and calcitonin gene-related peptide in the mucociliary defence of the rabbit maxillary sinus. Rhinology *25:* 89–93 (1987).

278 Messerklinger, W.: Über die Sekretströmung auf der Schleimhaut der oberen Luftwege. Z. Lar. Rhinol. Otol. *30:* 302–308 (1951).

279 Messerklinger, W.: Über periodische Veränderungen des Flimmerepithels der Luftwege durch Reizung des vegetativen Systems. Arch. Ohr-Nas.-KehlkHeilk. *167:* 345–349 (1955).

280 Messerklinger, W.: Flimmerepithel der Luftwege und vegetatives Nervensystem. Z. Lar. Rhinol. Otol. *35:* 3–27 (1956).

281 Messerklinger, W.: Die Schleimhaut der oberen Luftwege im Blickfeld neuerer Forschung. Arch. Ohr-Nas.-KehlkHeilk. *173:* 1–104 (1958).

282 Messerklinger, W.: Über die Drainage der menschlichen Nasennebenhöhlen unter normalen und pathologischen Bedingungen. 1. Mitteilung. Mschr. Ohrenheilk. Lar.-Rhinol. *100:* 56–68 (1966).

283 Messerklinger, W.: On the drainage of the normal frontal sinus of man. Acta oto-lar. *63:* 176–181 (1967).

284 Messerklinger, W.: Über die Drainage der menschlichen Nasennebenhöhlen unter normalen und pathologischen Bedingungen 2. Mitteilung. Mschr. Ohrenheilk. Lar.-Rhinol. *101:* 313–326 (1967).

285 Messerklinger, W.: Ist in allen menschlichen Stirnhöhlen das Prinzip des Sekrettransportes gleich? Arch. klin. exp. Ohr.-Nas.-KehlkHeilk. *189:* 317–326 (1967).

286 Messerklinger, W.: Die normalen Sekretwege in der Nase des Menschen. Arch. Ohr.-Nas.-KehlkHeil. *195:* 138–151 (1969).

287 Messerklinger, W.: Endoskopie der Nase und der Nebenhöhlen; in Berendes, Link, Zöllner, Hals-Nasen-Ohrenheilkunde in Praxis und Klinik, Band 1 (Thieme, Stuttgart 1977).

288 Messerklinger, W.: Endoscopy of the nose (Urban & Schwarzenberg, Baltimore 1978).

289 Miani, P.: Sul comportamento delle cilia vibratili della tuba di eustachio e della trachea sotto l'azione dei raggi X e dei raggi X del radium. Minerva otorhinolaring. *9:* 143–148 (1959).

290 Moreau, M.F.; Chretien, M.F.; Dubin, J.: Transposed ciliary microtubules in Kartagener's syndrome. A case report with electron microscopy of bronchial and nasal brushings. Acta cytol. *29:* 248–253 (1985).

291 Morgan, K.T.; Jiany, X.-Z.; Patterson, D.L.; Gross, E.A.: The nasal mucociliary apparatus; correlation of structure and function in the rat. Am. Rev. resp. Dis. *130:* 275–281 (1984).

292 Morgan, K.T.; Gross, E.A.; Patterson, D.L.: Distribution, progression, and recovery of acute formaldehyde-induced inhibition of nasal mucociliary function in F-334 rats. Toxicol. appl. Pharmacol. *86:* 448–456 (1986).

293 Morrow, P.E.: An evaluation of the physical properties of monodisperse and heterodisperse aerosols used in the assessment of bronchial function. Chest *80:* suppl., pp. 809–813 (1981).

294 Mostow, S.R.; Dreisin, R.B.; Manawadu, B.R.; Marc la Force, F.: Adverse effects of lidocaine and methylparaben on tracheal ciliary activity. Laryngoscope, St Louis *89:* 1697 (1979).

295 Müller, E.: Die Frühformen des Stimmlippenkarzinomes und deren Diagnose. Z. Lar. Rhinol. Otol. *35:* 174–183 (1956).

296 Müller, M.; Konietzko, N.; Adam, W.E.; Matthys, H.: Die mucociliare Clearance der Lunge; untersucht mit radioaktiv markiertem Schwefelkolloid. Klin. Wschr. *53:* 815–822 (1975).

297 Munkner, T.; Pedersen, M.: Lung scintigraphy in 22 patients with primary ciliary dyskinesia. Eur. J. resp. Dis. *64:* suppl., pp. 479–480 (1983).

298 Murakami, A.: Control of ciliary beat frequency in the gill of Mytilus. I. Activation of the lateral cilia by cyclic AMP II. Effects of saponin and Brij-58 on the lateral cilia. Comp. Biochem. Physiol. C Comp. Pharmacol. Toxicol. *86:* 273–287 (1987).

299 Mygind, N.: Nasal allergy (Blackwell, Oxford 1978).

300 Mygind, N.; Pedersen, M.; Nielsen, M.H.: Morphology of the upper airway epithelium; in Proctor, Andersen, The nose (Elsevier, Amsterdam 1982).

301 Mygind, N.; Pedersen, M.; Nielsen, M.H.: Primary and secondary ciliary dyskinesia. Acta oto-lar. *95:* 688–694 (1983).

302 Nakhosteen, J.A.; Zavala, D.C.: Atlas und Lehrbuch der flexiblen Bronchoskopie (Springer, Berlin 1983).

303 Negus, V.: The comparative anatomy and physiology of the nose and paranasal sinuses (Livingstone, Edinburgh 1958).

304 Newhouse, M.T.: Pathophysiology of dyskinetic cilia (Kartagener) syndrome; in Rensch, Mukustransport (Dustri, München 1980).

305 Nuutinen, J.; Kärja, J.; Karjalainen, P.: Measurements of impaired mucociliary activity in children. Eur. J. resp. Dis. *64:* suppl. 128, pp 454–456 (1983).

306 Nuutinen, J.: Activation of the nasal cilia. Rhinology *23:* 3–10 (1985).

307 Nuutinen, J.: Activation of the impaired nasal mucociliary function. Acta oto-lar. *99:* 605–609 (1985).

308 Nuutinen, J.: Activation of the impaired nasal mucociliary transport in children: preliminary report. Int. J. pediat. ORL *10:* 47–52 (1985).

309 Ogura, J.H.; Thawley, Cysts and tumors of the larynx; in Paparella, Shumrick, Oto-laryngology, vol. III (Saunders, Philadelphia 1980).

310 Ohashi, Y.; Nakai, Y.: Reduced ciliary action in chronic sinusitis. Acta oto-lar. suppl. 397, pp. 3–9 (1983).

311 Ohashi, Y.; Nakai, Y.: Functional and morphological pathology of chronic sinusitis mucous membrane. Acta oto-lar. suppl. 397, pp. 11–48 (1983).

312 Ohashi, Y.; Nakai, Y.; Zushi, K.; Muraoka, M.; Minowa, Y.; Harada, H.; Masutani, H.: Enhancement of ciliary action by a β-adrenergic stimulant. Acta oto-lar., suppl. 397, pp. 49–59 (1983).

313 Ohashi, Y.; Nakai, Y.: Mucociliary activities in fetal rabbits. Acta oto-lar. *97:* 351–358 (1984).

314 Ohashi, Y.; Nakai, Y.; Kihara, S.; Maruoka, K.; Ikeoka, H.; Uemura, Y.: The ciliary activity of the middle ear lining – functional and morphological observations. Auris nasus larynx *12:* suppl. 1, pp. 123–125 (1985).

315 Ohashi, Y.; Nakai, Y.; Ikeoka, H.; Koshimo, H.; Onoyama, Y.: Effects of irradiation on the ciliary activity of the eustachian tube and middle ear mucosa. Archs Oto-Rhino-Lar. *242:* 343–348 (1985).

316 Ohashi, Y.; Nakai, Y.; Kihara, S.: Ciliary activity of the middle ear lining in guinea pigs. Ann. Otol. *94:* 419–423 (1985).

317 Ohashi, Y.; Nakai, Y.; Kihara, S.; Ikeoka, H.; Takano, H.; Imoto, T.: Ciliary activity in patients with nasal allergies. Archs Oto-Rhino-Lar. *242:* 141–147 (1985).

318 Ohashi, Y.; Nakai, Y.; Koshimo, H.; Esaki, Y.: Ciliary activity in the in vitro tubo-tympanum. Archs Oto-Rhino-Lar. *243:* 317–319 (1986).

319 Ohashi, Y.; Nakai, Y.; Muraoka, M.: Abnormal mucociliary function in a mucocele of the maxillary antrum. Archs Oto-Rhino-Lar. *243:* 207–210 (1986).

320 Ohashi, Y.; Nakai, Y.; Ileoka, H.; Koshimo, H.; Esaki, Y.; Kato, S.: Effects of bacterial endotoxin on the ciliary activity in the in vitro eustachian tube. Archs Oto-Rhino-Lar. *244:* 88–90 (1987).

321 Ohashi, Y.; Nakai, Y.; Ikeoka, H.; Koshimo, H.; Esaki, Y.: Effects of bacterial endotoxin on the ciliary activity in the in vitro middle ear mucosa. Acta oto-lar. *104:* 495–499 (1987).

322 Ohi, M.; Sakakura, Y.; Murai, S.; Miyoshi, Y.: Effect of ipratropium bromide on nasal mucociliary transport. Rhinology *22:* 241–246 (1984).

323 Papanicolaou, G.N.: Degenerative changes in ciliated cells exfoliating from bronchial epithelium as a cytological criterion in the diagnosis of diseases of the lung. N.Y.S. J. Med. *56:* 2647 (1956).

324 Parker, G.S.; Mehlum, D.L.; Bea Bacher-Wetmore, M.S.; Ciliary dyskinesis: the immotile cilia syndrome. Laryngoscope St Louis *93:* 573 (1983).

325 Passali, D.; Bellussi, L.; Ciampoli Bianchi, M.; De Seta, E.: Experiences in the determination of nasal mucociliary transport time. Acta oto-lar. *97:* 319–323 (1984).

326 Passali, D.; Bianchi Ciampoli, M.: Normal values of mucociliary transport time in young subjects. Int. J. pediat. ORL *9:* 151–156 (1985).

327 Passali, D.; Bianchini-Ciampoli, M.; Volpino, P.: Influenza del fumo di sigaretta sul trasporto mucociliare nasale e tracheale. Riv. ital. ORL Audiol. Foniat. *4:* 530–535 (1985).

328 Patrick, G.; Stirling, C.; Measurement of mucociliary clearance from the trachea of conscious and anaesthetized rats. J. appl. Physiol. *42:* 451–455 (1977).

329 Pavelka, M.; Ronge, H.R.; Stockinger, G.: Vergleichende Untersuchungen am Trachealepithel verschiedener Säuger. Acta anat. *94:* 262–282 (1976).

330 Pavia, D.; Agnew, J.E.; Bateman, J.R.M.; Sheahan, N.F.; Knight, R.K.; Hendry, W.F.; Clarke, S.W.: Lung mucociliary clearance in patients with Young's syndrome. Chest *80:* suppl., pp. 892–895 (1981).

331 Pavia, D.; Sutton, P.P.; Lopez-Vidriero, M.T.; Angew, J.E.; Clarke, S.W.: Drug effects on mucociliary function. Eur. J. resp. Dis. *64:* suppl. 128, pp. 304–317 (1983).

332 Pedersen, M.; Rebbe, H.: Absence of arms in the axoneme of immotile human spermatozoa. Biol. Reprod. *12:* 541–544 (1975).

333 Pedersen, M.; Morkassel, E.; Nielsen, M.H.; Mygind, N.: Kartagener's syndrome: preliminary report on cilia structure, function, and upper airway symptoms. Chest *80:* suppl., pp. 858–860 (1981).

334 Pedersen, M.; Sakakura, Y.; Winther, B.; Brofeldt, S.; Mygind, N.: Nasal mucociliary transport, number of ciliated cells and beating pattern in naturally acquired common colds. Eur. J. resp. Dis. *64:* suppl. 128, pp. 355–364 (1983).

335 Pemsingh, R.S.; Atwal, O.S.; McPherson, R.B.: Atypical cilia in a ciliated cyst of the parathyroid glands of dogs exposed to ozone. Exp. Pathol. *28:* 105–110 (1985).

336 Perry, R.J.; Smaldone, G.C.: Does prolonged bronchodilator therapy increase mucociliary clearance and lung permeability in normal humans. Am. Rev. resp. Dis. *132:* suppl. 4, A 49 (1986).

337 Petruson, B.; Hansson, H.A.; Karlsson, G.: Structural and functional aspects of cells in the nasal mucociliary system. Archs Otolar. *110:* 576–581 (1984).

338 Philipson, K.: Radioisotope labelling of aerosols for the study of lung function. Chest *80:* suppl., pp. 818–820 (1981).

339 Phillips, F.L.: The role of ciliated epithelium in sinusitis. Ann. Otol. *35:* 709–716 (1926).

340 Proctor, D.F.: Measurement of mucociliary activity in man. Ann. Otol. *78:* 518–531 (1969).

341 Proctor, D.F.; Andersen, I.: The nose, upper airway physiology and the atmospheric environment (Elsevier, Amsterdam, 1982).

342 Proctor, D.F.: Nasal mucous transport and our ambient air. Laryngoscope, St Louis *93:* 58–62 (1983).

343 Proetz, A.W.: Studies of nasal cilia in the living mammal. Ann. Otol. *42:* 778–785 (1933).

344 Proetz, A.W.; Pfingsten, M.: Ciliated nasal epithelium: its culture in vitro, preliminary report. Ann. Otol. *45:* 400–409 (1936).

345 Proetz, A.W.: Applied physiology of the nose (Annals Publishing, St. Louis 1953).

346 Puchelle, A.; Aug, F.; Pham, Q.T.; Betrand, A.: Comparison of three methods for measuring nasal mucociliary activity. Acta oto-lar. *91:* 297 (1981).

347 Puchelle, A.; Tournier, J.M.; Petit, A.; Zahm, J.M.; Lauque, D.; Vidailhet, M.; Sadoul, P.: The frog palate for studying mucus transport velocity and mucociliary frequency. Eur. J. resp. Dis. *64:* suppl. 128, pp. 293–303 (1983).

348 Puchelle, E.; Zahm, J.M.; Tournier, J.M.: Cilio-inhibitory effect of human leucocyte elastase; influence of tris buffer. Am. Rev. resp. Dis. *132:* suppl. 4, A 73 (1986).

349 Pullan, C.R.; Roberton, D.M.; Milner, A.D.; Robinson, G.; Perkins, A.; Campbell, A.C.: Investigation of children with abnormal cilia, Eur. J. resp. Dis. *64:* suppl. 128, pp. 466–469 (1983).

350 Purkinje, J.E.; Valentin, G.G.: Entdeckung continuierlicher und durch Wimpernhaare erzeugter Flimmerbewegungen als ein allgemeines Phänomen in der Klasse der Amphibien, Vögel und Säugetiere. Müllers Arch. Anat. Physiol. *5:* 391–409 (1834).

351 Quinlan, M.F.; Salman, S.D.; Swift, D.S.; Wagner, H.N.; Proctor, D.F.: Measurement of mucociliary function in man. Am. Rev. resp. Dis. *99:* 12–23 (1969).

352 Rautiainen, M.; Collan, Y.; Nuutinen, J.: A method for measuring the orientation ('beat direction') of respiratory cilia. Archs Oto-Rhino-Lar. *243:* 265–268 (1986).

353 Rautiainen, M.; Collan, Y.; Kärjä, J.; Nuutinen. J.: Artifacts in ultrastructure of respiratory cilia caused by various fixation procedures and different types of handling. ORL *49:* 193–198 (1987).

354 Reimer, A.; Hakansson, C.H.; Mercke, U.; Toremalm, N.G.: The mucociliary activity of the upper respiratory tract. Acta oto-lar. *83:* 491–497 (1977).

355 Reimer, A.; Toremalm, N.G.: The mucociliary activity of the upper respiratory tract. Acta oto-lar. *86:* 283–288 (1978).

356 Reimer, A.; Mecklenburg, C. von; Toremalm, N.G.: The mucociliary activity of the upper respiratory tract III. A functional and morphological study on human and animal material with special reference to maxillary sinus disease. Acta oto-lar., suppl. 355, pp. 1–20 (1978).

357 Reimer, A.; Klementsson, K.; Ursing, J.; Wretlind, B.: The mucociliary activity of the respiratory tract. Acta oto-lar. *90:* 462–469 (1980).

358 Reimer, A.; Hubermann, D.; Klementsson, K.; Toremalm, N.G.: The mucociliary activity of the respiratory tract. Acta oto-lar. *91:* 139–148 (1981).

359 Reimer, A.: The effect of carbon dioxide on the activity of cilia. Acta oto-lar. *103:* 156–160 (1987).

360 Reissig, M.; Bang, B.G.; Bang, F.B.: Ultrastructure of the mucociliary interface in the nasal mucosa of the children. Am. Rev. resp. Dis. *117:* 327–341 (1978).

361 Rhodin, J.: Ultrastructure of the tracheal ciliated mucosa in rat and man. Ann. Otol. *68:* 964–974 (1959).

362 Rhodin, J.: Ultrastructure and function of the human tracheal mucosa. Am. Rev. resp. Dis. *93:* suppl., pp. 1–15 (1966).

363 Richter, H.G.: Das rasterelektronenmikroskopische Bild der Trachealschleimhaut nach translaryngealer intratrachealer Langzeitintubation. Lar. Rhinol. Otol. *61:* 90–92 (1982).

364 Roessler, F.: Geeignete Methoden zur Untersuchung primärer Zilienfunktionsstörungen. Zentbl. Hals-Nasen-Ohrenheilk. *132:* 787–788 (1986).

365 Rossman, C.M.; Forrest, J.; Newhouse, M.: Motile cilia in immotile cilia syndrome. Lancet *i:* 1360 (1980).

366 Rossman, C.M.; Forrest, J.B.; Lee, R.M.K.W.; Newhouse, A.F.; Newhouse, M.T.: The dyskinetic cilia syndrome. Chest *80:* suppl., pp. 860–865 (1981).

367 Rossman, C.M.; Lee, R.M.K.W.; Forrest, J.B.; Newhouse, M.T.: Nasal ciliary ultrastructure and function in patients with primary ciliary dyskinesia compared with that in normal subjects and in subjects with various respiratory diseases. Am. Rev. resp. Dis. *129:* 161–167 (1984).

368 Roth, Y.; Ostfeld, E.: Ciliary beat frequency of human middle ear mucosa measured in vitro. J. Lar. Otol. *98:* 853–856 (1984).

369 Roth, Y.; Kimhi, Y.; Edery, H.: Ciliary motility in brain ventricular system and trachea of hamsters. Brain Res. *330:* 291–297 (1985).

370 Ruckes, J.; Hollstein, H.: Morphologische Befunde an Trachea und Bronchien nach Betatronbestrahlung von Bronchialkarzinomen. Strahlentherapie *136:* 515–520 (1968).

371 Rühle, K.H.; Köhler, D.; Fischer, J.; Matthys, H.: Measurement of mucociliary clearance with ^{99}Tc tagget erythrocytes. Prog. Resp. Res., vol. 11, pp. 117–126 (Karger, Basel 1979).

372 Rühle, K.H.; Vastag, E.; Köhler, D.; Matthys, H.: Ziliarer und nichtziliarer Partikeltransport; in Rügheimer, Intubation, Tracheotomie, bronchopulmonale Infektion (Springer, Berlin 1983).

373 Russo, K.J.; Palmer, D.W.; Beste, D.J.: Radioisotopic measurement of the velocity of tracheal mucus. Otolaryngol Head Neck Surg. *93:* 217–220 (1985).

374 Rutland, J.; Cole, P.J.: Non-invasive sampling of nasal cilia for measurement of beat frequency and study of ultrastructure. Lancet *ii:* 564 (1980).

375 Rutland, J.; Cole, P.J.: Ciliary dyskinesia. Lancet *ii:* 859 (1980).

376 Rutland, J.; Griffin, W.M.; Cole, P.J.: Nasal brushing and measurement of ciliary beat frequency. Chest *80:* suppl., pp. 865–867 (1981).

377 Rutland, J.; Griffin, W.M.; Cole, P.J.: Human ciliary beat frequency in epithelium from intrathoracic and extrathoracic airways. Am. Rev. resp. Dis. *125:* 100–105 (1982).

378 Rutland, J.; Cox, T.; Dewar, A.; Rehahn, M.; Cole, P.J.: Relationship between dynein arms and ciliary motility in Kartagener's syndrome. Eur. J. resp. Dis. *64:* suppl. 128, pp. 470–472 (1983).

379 Rutland, J.; Penketh, A.; Griffin, W.; Hodson, M.; Batten, J.; Cole, P.J.: Lack of effect of cystic fibrosis serum on human ciliary motility. Eur. J. resp. Dis. *64:* suppl. 128, pp. 451–453 (1983).

380 Rylander, R.: Current techniques to measure alterations in the ciliary activity of intact respiratory epithelium. Am. Rev. resp. Dis. *93:* suppl., pp. 67–72 (1966).

381 Sackner, M.A.; Rosen, M.J.; Wanner, A.: Estimation of tracheal mucous velocity by bronchofiberscopy. J. appl. Physiol. *34:* 495–499 (1973).

382 Sackner, M.A.; Reinhart, M.; Arkin, B.: Effects of beclomethasone dipropionate on tracheal mucus velocity. Am. Rev. resp. Dis. *115:* 1069–1077 (1977).

383 Sadé, J.; Eliezer, N.; Silberberg, A.; Nevo, A.C.: The role of mucus in transport by cilia. Am. Rev. resp. Dis. *102:* 48–52 (1970).

384 Sadé, J.; Eliezer, N.: Secretory otilis media and the nature of the mucociliary system. Acta oto-lar. *70:* 351–357 (1970).

385 Sadoul, P.; Puchelle, E.; Zahm, M.J.; Jacquot, J.; Aug, F.; Pulu, J.M.: Effect of terbutalin on mucociliary transport and sputum properties in chronic bronchitis. Chest *80:* suppl., pp. 885–888 (1981).

386 Sakakura, Y.; Sasaki, Y.; Hornick, R.B.; Togo, Y.; Schwartz, A.R.; Wagner, H.N.; Proctor, D.F.: Mucociliary function during experimentally induced rhinovirus infection in man. Ann. Otol. *82:* 203–211 (1973).

387 Sakakura, Y.; Ukai, K.; Majima, Y.; Murai, S.; Harada, T.; Miyoshi, Y.: Nasal mucociliary clearance under various conditions. Acta oto-lar. *96:* 167–173 (1983).

388 Sakakura, Y.: Changes of mucociliary function during colds. Eur. J. resp. Dis. *64:* suppl. 128, pp. 348–354 (1983).

389 Sakakura, Y.; Ukai, K.; Yamagiwa, M.; Murai, S.; Hori, M.; Miyoshi, Y.: Nasal mucociliary function in man. J. Otolaryngol. Jpn. *83:* 1592–1597 (1980).

390 Sakakura, Y.; Majima, Y.; Saida, S.; Ukai, K.; Mioshi, Y.: Reversibility of reduced mucociliary clearance in chronic sinusitis. Clin. Otolaryngol. *10:* 79–83 (1985).

391 Saketkhoo, K.; Yergin, B.M.; Januszkiewicz, A.; Kovitz, K.; Sackner, M.A.: The effect of nasal decongestants on nasal mucous velocity. Am. Rev. resp. Dis. *118:* 251–254 (1978).

392 Santa Cruz, R.; Lauda, J.; Hirsch, J.; Sackner, M.A.: Tracheal mucous velocity in man and patients with obstructive lung disease. Effects of terbutaline. Am. Rev. resp. Dis. *109:* 458–463 (1974).

393 Satir, P.: Studies on cilia II: Examination of the distal region of the ciliary shaft and the role of the filaments in motility. J. Cell Biol. *26:* 805–834 (1965).

394 Satir, P.: How cilia move. Scient. Am. *231:* 45–52 (1974).

395 Satir, P.; Wais-Steider, J.; Lebduska, S.; Nasr, A.; Avolio, J.: The mechanochemical cycle of the dynein arm. Cell Motility *1:* 303–327 (1981).

396 Scott, G.B.D.: A quantitative study of microscopical changes in the epithelium and

subepithelial tissue of the laryngeal folds, sinus and saccule. Clin. Otolaryngol. *1:* 257–264 (1976).

397 Sharpey, W.: On a peculiar motion excited in fluids by the surfaces of certain animals. Edinb. med. surg. J. *34:* 113–122 (1830).

398 Shih, C.K.; Litt, M.; Khan, M.A.; Wolf, D.P.: Effect of nondialyzable solids concentration and viscoelasticity on ciliary transport of tracheal mucus. Am. Rev. resp. Dis. *115:* 989–995 (1977).

399 Simon, J.; Drettner, B.; Jung, B.: Messung des Schleimhauttransportes in menschlichen Nasen mit ^{51}Cr-markierten Harzkügelchen. Acta oto-lar. *83:* 378–390 (1977).

400 Sleigh, M.A.: Some aspects of the comparative physiology of cilia. Am. Rev. resp. Dis. *93:* suppl., pp. 17–31 (1966).

401 Sleigh, M.A.: Cilia and flagella (Academic Press, London 1974).

402 Sleigh, M.A.: Ciliary function in mucus transport. Chest *80:* suppl. 6, pp. 791–795 (1981).

403 Sleigh, M.A.: Primary ciliary dyskinesia. Lancet *ii:* 476 (1981).

404 Sleigh, M.A.: Discussion to: Rossman et al. The dyskinetic cilia syndrome. Chest *80:* suppl., p. 864 (1981).

405 Sleigh, M.A.: Ciliary function in transport of mucus. Eur. J. resp. Dis. *64:* suppl. 128, pp. 287–292 (1983).

406 Sugar, J.; Farago, L.: Ultrastructure of laryngeal precanceroses. Acta oto-lar. *62:* 319–332 (1966).

407 Surjan, L.; Bajtai, A.: The role of scanning electron microscopy in the diagnosis of human laryngeal cancer. Acta oto-lar. *99:* 236–238 (1985).

408 Sutton, P.P.; Pavia, D.; Bateman, J.R.M.; Clarke, S.W.: The effect of oral aminophylline on lung mucociliary clearance in man. Chest *80:* suppl., pp. 889–892 (1981).

409 Svedbergh, B.; Jonsson, V.; Afzelius, B.A.: Immotile-cilia syndrome and the cilia of the eye. Graefes Arch. Ophthal. *215:* 265–272 (1981).

410 Swain, H.L.: Ciliated epithelium and other protective agencies. Ann. Otol. *33:* 1299–1306 (1924).

411 Schwab, W.: Diskussionsbemerkung. Arch. Ohr-Nas.-KehlkHeilk. *167:* 349 (1955).

412 Stammberger, H.; Messerklinger W.: Endoscopic diagnosis, surgery and treatment of paranasal sinus mycoses (Compliments of Karl Storz, Tuttlingen 1984).

413 Stanley, P.J.; Griffin, W.M.; Wilson, R.: Effect of betamethasone and betamethasone with neomycine nasal drops on human nasal mucociliary clearance and ciliary beat frequency. Thorax *40:* 607–612 (1985).

414 Stell, P.M.; Gregory, I.; Watt, J.: Techniques for demonstrating the epithelial lining of the larynx. J. Lar. Otol. *86:* 589–594 (1972).

415 Stell, P.M.; Gregory, I.; Watt, J.: Morphometry of the epithelial lining of the human larynx. I. The glottis. Clin. Otolaryngol. *3:* 13–20 (1978).

416 Stell, P.M.; Gregory, I.; Watt, J.: Morphology of the human larynx. II. The subglottis. Clin. Otolaryngol. *5:* 389–395 (1980).

417 Stenfors, L.E.; Hellstrom, S.; Albiin, N.: Middle ear clearance. Ann. Otol. *94:* suppl. 120, pp. 30–31 (1985).

418 Stewart, W.C.: Weight carrying capacity and excitability of excised ciliated epithelium. Am. J. Physiol. *152:* 1–12 (1948).

419 Stuart-Harris, C.H.: Respiratory viruses, ciliated epithelium, and bronchitis. Am. Rev. resp. Dis. *93:* suppl., pp. 151–155 (1966).

420 Sturgess, J.M.; Chao, J.; Wong, J.; Aspin, N.; Turner, J.A.P.: Cilia with defective radial spokes; a cause of human respiratory disease. New Engl. J. Med. *300:* 53–56 (1979).

421 Sturgess, J.M.; Chao, J.; Turner, J.A.P.: Transposition of ciliary microtubules. New Engl. J. Med. *303:* 318–322 (1980).

422 Takasaka, T.; Sato, M.; Onodera, A.: Atypical cilia of the human nasal mucosa. Ann. Otol. *89:* 37–45 (1980).

423 Takasaka, T.; Kawamoto, K.: Mucociliary dysfunction in experimental otitis media with effusion. Am. J. Otolaryngol. Head Neck Surg. *6:* 232–236 (1985).

424 Tanaka, T.; Benedek, G.B.: Measurement of the velocity of bloodflow (in vivo) using a fiber optic catheter and optical mixing spectroscopy. Appl. Optics *14:* 189–196 (1975).

425 Terrier, G.: L'épreuve du transport muco-ciliaire coloré dans le sinus maxillaire. Aktuelle Probl. ORL *7:* 164–167 (1984).

426 Theopold, H.-M.; Jahnke, V.; Schinko I.: Zur Feinstruktur der Zilien beim Kartagener-Syndrom. Lar. Rhinol. Otol. *63:* 33–40 (1984).

427 Toremalm, N.G.: Air-flow patterns and ciliary activity in the trachea after tracheotomy. Acta oto-lar. *53:* 442–454 (1961).

428 Toremalm, N.G.; Hakansson, C.H.; Mercke, U.; Dahlerns, B.: Mucociliary wave pattern. Acta oto-lar. *78:* 247–252 (1974).

429 Toremalm, N.G.; Mercke, U.; Reimer, A.: The mucociliary activity of the upper respiratory tract. Rhinology *13:* 113–120 (1975).

430 Toremalm, N.G.; Hakansson, C.H.; Mercke, U.; Reimer, A.: Intra- and extracellular activities of ciliated cells. Acta oto-lar. *83:* 34–38 (1977).

431 Toremalm, N.G.: The mucociliary apparatus. Rhinology *21:* 197–202 (1983).

432 Toremalm, N.G.: Aerodynamics and mucociliary function of upper airways. Eur. J. resp. Dis. *66:* suppl. 139, pp. 54–56 (1985).

433 Torikata, C.; Takenchi, H.; Yamaguchi, H.; Kageyama, K.: Abnormal cilia in bronchial mucosa – case reports of non-smoking women with bronchiogenic carcinomas and an experimental model in guinea-pigs. Virchows Arch. A. Path. Anat. Histol. *371:* 121–129 (1976).

434 Tos, M.: Goblet cells and glands in the nose and paranasal sinuses; in Proctor, Andersen, The nose (Elsevier Biomedical Press, Amsterdam 1982).

435 Tos, M.: Diskussionsbemerkung bei Pedersen, M. u. MA. Eur. J. resp. Dis. *64:* suppl. 128, pp. 355–364 (1983).

436 Treeck, H.H.: Die Ultrastruktur der Grenzzone zwischen respiratorischem Epithel und nicht verhornendem Plattenepithel der Plica vocalis beim Menschen. Arch. Ohr-Nas.-KehlkHeilk. *207:* 554–555 (1974).

437 Tremble, G.E.: Diskussionsbemerkung bei Hilding A.C. Ciliary streaming through the larynx and distribution of laryngeal epithelium. Laryngoscope, St Louis *66:* 1362–1363 (1956).

438 Tremble, G.E.: Milestones in research of upper respiratory cilia. Arch. oto-lar. *75:* 346 (1962).

439 Tumarkin, A.: Stereocilia versus kinocilia. Part I: In the acoustic sensor. J. Lar. Otol. *100:* 1009–1018 (1986); Part II: In the vestibular sensor. J. Lar. Otol. *100:* 1107–1014 (1986).

440 Tyrell, D.A.J.: Discussion on Symposium Durham 1965. Am. Rev. resp. Dis. *93:* suppl. 83 (1966).

441 UICC: TNM-Atlas (Springer, Berlin 1985).

442 Ukai, K.; Bang, B.G.; Bang, F.B.: Effect of SO_2 exposure on nasal mucociliary clearance in intact chickens. Auris Nasus Larynx, Tokyo *10:* 97–107 (1983).

443 Ukai, K.; Bang, B.G.; Bang, F.B.: Effect of infection and SO_2-exposure on nasal and paranasal mucociliary clearance in intact chickens. Archs Oto-Rhino-Lar. *239:* 1–6 (1984).

444 Ukai, K.; Bang, B.G.; Bang, F.B.: Effect of mechanical stimulation on mucociliary clearance of chicken sinus. Rhinology *22:* 35–43 (1984).

445 Ukai, K.; Sakakura, Y.; Saida, S.: Interaction between mucociliary transport and the ciliary beat of chicken nasal mucosa. Archs Oto-Rhino-Lar. *242:* 225–231 (1985).

446 Ukai, K.; Sakakura, Y.; Mioshi, A.; Uchida, Y.: Pathophysiological condition of the nose of asthmatic children with subclinical allergy. Rhinology *24:* 133–140 (1986).

447 Urban, J.: Die Wirkung des Histamins auf den Sekrettransport in der menschlichen Nase. Arch. klin. exp. Ohren-Nasen-KehlkHeilk. *189:* 327–336 (1967).

448 Veerman, A.J.P.; van der Baan, A.; Weltevreden, E.F.; Leene, W.; Feenstra, L.: Cilia: Immotile, dyskinetic, dysfunctional. Lancet *ii:* 266 (1980).

449 Veerman, A.J.P.; van Delden, L.; Feenstra, L.; Leene, W.: The immotile cilia syndrome: phase contrast light microscopy, scanning and transmission electron microscopy. Pediatrics *65:* 698–702 (1980).

450 Verdugo, P.; Rumery, R.E.; Tam, P.Y.: Hormonal control of oviductal ciliary activity: effects of prostaglandins. Fertil. Steril. *33:* 193–198 (1980).

451 Verdugo, P.: Ca^{2+}-dependent hormonal stimulation of ciliary activity. Nature *283:* 764–765 (1980).

452 Verdugo, P.; Johnson, N.T.; Tam, P.Y.: β-Adrenergic stimulation of respiratory ciliary activity. J. appl. Physiol. *48:* 868–871 (1980).

453 Voss, R.; Reichborn-Kjennerud, S.; Abeler, V.; Reith, A.: Development of brush cytology for detection of metaplastic and dysplastic nasal mucosa lesions. Acta otolar. *101:* 299–305 (1986).

454 Wacker, D.F.; Howe, M.L.: Middle ear cilia activity as a determinant of tympanostomy tube placement. Otolaryngol. Head Neck Surg. *95:* 434–437 (1986).

455 Waite, D.A.; Wakefield, J.; Mackay, J.B.; Ross, I.T.: Mucociliary transport and ultrastructural abnormalities in polynesian bronchiectasis. Chest *80:* suppl., pp. 896–898 (1981).

456 Wanner, A.: Alteration of tracheal mucociliary transport in airway disease. Chest *80:* suppl., pp. 867–870 (1981).

457 Wanner, A.: Allergic mucociliary dysfunction. Laryngoscope, St Louis *93:* 68–70 (1983).

458 Warwick, W.J.: Mechanisms of mucous transport. Eur. J. resp. Dis. *64:* suppl. 128, pp. 162–167 (1983).

459 Watanabe, Y.; Okuda, M.: How can we detect patients with immotile cilia syndrome? Eur. J. resp. Dis. *64:* suppl. 128, pp. 473–475 (1983).

460 Watanabe, Y.; Okuda, M.: Ultrastructural study of immotile cilia syndrome. Rhinology *22:* 193–199 (1984).

461 Weiss, T.; Dorow, P.; Felix, R.: Effects of a beta adrenergic drug and a secretolytic

agent on regional mucociliary clearance in patients with cold. Chest *80:* suppl., pp. 881–885 (1981).

462 Werner, W.; Privara, M.: Rasterelektronenmikroskopische Studie zum Oberflächen-relief der Schleimhaut von Larynx und Trachea. HNO-Praxis, Leipzig *1/2:* 24–29 (1976).

463 Westhofen, M.; Lee, Y.; Herberhold, C.: Zur Biologie imolantierter homologer Tra-chealsegmente. Archs Oto-Rhino-Lar., suppl. II, p. 246 (1984).

464 Wetmore, R.F.; Brown, D.T.; Litt, M.; Potsic, W.P.: Human tracheal mucin: a pre-liminary study of physicochemical properties and mucociliary transport. Otolaryn-gol. Head Neck Surg. *91:* 509–515 (1983).

465 White, B.L.; Catlin, F.I.; Stenback, W.A.; Hawkins, E.D.; Seilheimer, D.K.: The immotile cilia syndrome, one cause of persistent upper respiratory tract infection. Int. J. pediat. ORL *2:* 337–346 (1980).

466 Widdicombe, J.G.; Wells, U.M.: Airway secretion; in Proctor, Andersen, The nose, upper airway physiology and atmospheric environment (Elsevier Biomedical Press, Amsterdam 1982).

467 Wilson, D.W.; Plopper, C.G.; Dungworth, D.L.: The response of the macaque tra-cheobronchial epithelium to acute ozone injury. Am. J. Pathol. *116:* 193–206 (1984).

468 Wilson, R.; Roberts, D.; Cole, P.: Effect of bacterial products on human ciliary function. Thorax *40:* 125–131 (1985).

469 Winther, B.; Brofeldt, S.; Christensen, B.; Mygind, N.: Light and scanning electron microscopy of nasal biopsy material from patients with naturally acquired common cold. Acta oto-lar. *97:* 309–318 (1984).

470 Wisseman, C.L.; Simel, D.L.; Spock, A.; Shelburne, J.D.: The prevalence of abnor-mal cilia in normal pediatric lungs. Arch. Pathol. Lab. Med. *105:* 552–555 (1981).

471 Wolff, R.K.; Muggenburg, B.A.: Comparison of two methods of measuring tracheal mucus velocity in anaesthesized beagle dogs. Am. Rev. resp. Dis. *120:* 137–142 (1979).

472 Wright, G.W.: Effects of industrial dust on ciliated epithelium. Am. Rev. resp. Dis. *93:* suppl., pp. 103–107 (1966).

473 Yager, J.; Chen, Tzeng-Ming; Dulfano, M.J.: Measurement of frequency of ciliary beats of human respiratory epithelium. Chest *73:* 627–633 (1978).

474 Yates, A.L.: Methods of estimating the activity of the ciliated epithelium within the sinuses. J. Laryngol. *39:* 554 (1924).

475 Yeates, D.B.; Aspin, N.; Levison, H.; Jones, M.T.; Bryan, A.C.: Mucociliary tracheal transport rates in man. J. appl. Physiol. *39:* 487–495 (1975).

476 Yeates, D.B.; Matthys, H.: Diskussionszusammenfassung. Workshop Miami/USA 1981. Chest *80:* suppl., p. 922 (1981).

477 Yergin, B.M.; Sakethkhoo, K.; Michaelson, E.D.; Serafini, S.M.; Kovitz, K.; Sack-ner, M.: A roentgenographic method for measuring nasal mucous velocity. J. appl. Physiol. *44:* 964–968 (1978).

478 Zaitsu, Y.: Laryngeal epithelium and mucous movement. Jap. J. Anest. *26:* 267–271 (1977).

479 Zilliacus, W.: Die Ausbreitung der verschiedenen Epithelarten im menschlichen Kehlkopf und eine neue Methode dieselbe festzustellen. Anat. Anz. *26:* 371–376 (1905).

Subject Index